# Brain Metastasis

# Brain Metastasis
## *A Multidisciplinary Approach*

*Edited by*

## Lawrence R. Kleinberg, MD
Associate Professor
Department of Radiation Oncology
The Johns Hopkins University School of Medicine
Baltimore, Maryland

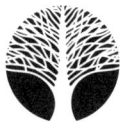

**demos**MEDICAL

New York

*Acquisitions Editor:* R. Craig Percy
*Cover Design:* A Good Thing, Inc.
*Copyeditor:* Tamara S. Cornelison
*Compositor:* TypeWriting
*Printer:* Malloy Lithographing

Visit our website at www.demosmedpub.com

Medicine is an ever-changing science. Research and clinical experience are continually expanding our knowledge, in particular our understanding of proper treatment and drug therapy. The authors, editors, and publisher have made every effort to ensure that all information in this book is in accordance with the state of knowledge at the time of production of the book. Nevertheless, the authors, editors, and publisher are not responsible for errors or omissions or for any consequences from application of the information in this book and make no warranty, express or implied, with respect to the contents of the publication. Every reader should examine carefully the package inserts accompanying each drug and should carefully check whether the dosage schedules mentioned therein or the contraindications stated by the manufacturer differ from the statements made in this book. Such examination is particularly important with drugs that are either rarely used or have been newly released on the market.

**Library of Congress Cataloging-in-Publication Data**

Brain metastasis : a multidisciplinary approach / edited by Lawrence R. Kleinberg.
   p. ; cm.
 Includes bibliographic references and index.
 ISBN-13: 978-1-933864-43-3 (hardcover : alk. paper)
 ISBN-10: 1-933864-43-5 (hardcover : alk. paper)
 1. Brain—Cancer. 2. Metastasis. I. Kleinberg, Lawrence R.
 [DNLM: 1. Brain Neoplasms—secondary. WL 358 B8131 2009]
 RC280.B7B684 2009
 616.99'481—dc22

                             2008024913

Special discounts on bulk quantities of Demos Medical Publishing books are available to corporations, professional associations, pharmaceutical companies, health care organizations, and other qualifying groups. For details, please contact:

Special Sales Department
Demos Medical Publishing
386 Park Avenue South, Suite 301
New York, NY 10016
Phone: 800–532–8663 or 212–683–0072
Fax: 212–683–0118
Email: orderdept@demosmedpub.com

Made in the United States of America

08 09 10 11   5 4 3 2 1

# Contents

# Preface

Although aggressive therapy of metastatic disease was previously thought to be of limited benefit compared with the associated cost and toxicities, new uses of older therapies and new treatments better targeted at metastatic disease have resulted in improved survival and quality of life for many patients. This has been made possible not only by the development of better agents and better understanding of potential uses, but also by the development of better management strategies for toxicities that make these agents much more palatable for patients. In addition, local therapies such as intensive radiation techniques and surgery are more often used even in palliative situations where they may have little impact on survival, a phenomenon driven by the growing recognition of the importance to patients of therapies that may address important quality of life concerns.

For all these reasons, radiosurgery for brain metastasis presents many advantages when used appropriately with selected patients with well-defined goals, and has become an attractive and viable option for oncologists and patients. In patients with limited disease in the brain and controlled disease elsewhere in the body, survival can be improved by more effective treatment of gross brain metastasis with radiosurgery. Under other circumstances, when prolonging survival may be questionable because of the likelihood of systemic progression, radiosurgery can be used to help prevent tumor-related injury of brain function and to maintain quality of life even after failure of whole-brain radiotherapy. Finally, radiosurgery can be used as an alternative to whole-brain radiotherapy, perhaps improving quality of life outcome by avoiding the potential, negative side effects of whole-brain radiotherapy.

Better use of systemic therapy is also making an important difference. In many early cases of breast or lung cancer, such treatment improves survival—presumably because it actually eliminates (in some patients) existing but undetected micrometastatic disease. In situations where cancer is more advanced and beyond cure, the value of systemic therapy, which can result in tumor response or delayed progression, has demonstrably improved short- and medium-term survival and improved quality of life.

As many systemic agents and biologic drugs may not penetrate the blood brain barrier well, the need for aggressive management of brain metastasis may increase. Brain lesions may continue to progress, even as the threat from tumor elsewhere in the body is successfully contained by systemic therapy. When viewed realistically, systemic therapy may be ineffectual in patients with advanced disease and poor performance status who may not be well served by these more intense, toxic, and costly approaches. Other patients, however, who in a prior era were told to go home to get their affairs in order, are now well served by such approaches and may look forward to living longer while meeting quality of life goals. This work focuses on a comprehensive approach to application of these principles for patients where metastasis has spread to the brain.

Lawrence R. Kleinberg

# Acknowledgments

I would like to express appreciation for the administrative support and assistance provided by Debbie Huesman and gratitude for the continued invaluable support of my wife, Allyn, and my daughter, Lauren.

# Contributors

**Laurie E. Blach, MD**
Attending Physician
Department of Radiation Oncology
Mt. Sinai Medical Center
Miami Beach, Florida
*Chapter 5: Radiosurgery for Brain
   Metastases*

**Jaishri Blakeley, MD**
Assistant Professor
Department of Neurology
The Johns Hopkins University
   School of Medicine
Baltimore, Maryland
*Chapter 1: Neurologic
   Manifestations of Brain
   Metastases: Recognition,
   Evolution, and Management*

**Sammie Coy, PhD**
Physicist
Gamma Knife Department
Miami Neuroscience Center
Coral Gables, Florida
*Chapter 5: Radiosurgery for Brain
   Metastases*

**Erin M. Dunbar, MD**
Assistant Professor
Department of Neurosurgery
University of Florida
Gainesville, Florida
*Chapter 7: Chemotherapy for Brain
   Metastasis: What We Know
   and What We Don't*

**James L. Frazier, MD**
Resident
Department of Neurosurgery
The Johns Hopkins University
   School of Medicine
Baltimore, Maryland
*Chapter 4: Surgical Management of
   Intracranial Metastases*

**Lawrence R. Kleinberg, MD**
Associate Professor
Department of Radiation Oncology
The Johns Hopkins University
   School of Medicine
Baltimore, Maryland
*Chapter 6: The Role of Targeted
   Therapy Without Whole-brain
   Radiotherapy*
*Chapter 9: Radiosurgry for Spinal
   Tumors*

**Jonathan P.S. Knisely, MD, FRCPC**
Associate Professor
Department of Therapeutic
    Radiology
Yale University School of Medicine
and Yale Cancer Center
New Haven, Connecticut
*Chapter 2: Radiation Therapy for
    Brain Metastases*
*Chapter 3: Prognosis of Patients
    with Brain Metastases Who
    Undergo Radiation Therapy*

**Jessica Kraker, MD**
Resident
Department of Neurology
University of Maryland
Baltimore, Maryland
*Chapter 1: Neurologic
    Manifestations of Brain
    Metastases: Recognition,
    Evolution, and Management*

**Michael Lim, MD**
Assistant Professor
Department of Neurosurgery
The Johns Hopkins University
    School of Medicine
Baltimore, Maryland
*Chapter 4: Surgical Management of
    Intracranial Metastases*

**Daniele Rigamonti, MD**
Professor
Director of Stereotactic
    Radiosurgery
Departments of Neurogsurgery,
    Radiosurgery, and Oncology
The Johns Hopkins University
    School of Medicine
Baltimore, Maryland
*Chapter 6: The Role of Targeted
    Therapy Without Whole-brain
    Radiotherapy*

**Ori Shokek, MD, BS**
Instructor
Department of Radiation Oncology
The Johns Hopkins University
    School of Medicine
Baltimore, Maryland
*Chapter 9: Radiosurgery for Spinal
    Tumors*

**Jon D. Weingart, MD**
Associate Professor
Department of Neurosurgery
The Johns Hopkins University
    School of Medicine
Baltimore, Maryland
*Chapter 4: Surgical Management of
    Intracranial Metastases*

**Stepanie E. Weiss, MD**
Attending Physician and Instructor
Department of Radiation Oncology
Brigham and Women's Hospital
Dana Farber Cancer Institute
Harvard Medical School
Boston, Massachusetts
*Chapter 8: Supportive Care:
    Controlling Symptoms of
    Brain Metastasis and
    Diminishing the Toxicities of
    Treatment*

**Aizik Loft Wolf, MD**
Director
Gamma Knife Department
Miami Neuroscience Center
Coral Gables, Florida
*Chapter 5: Radiosurgery for Brain
    Metastases*

**James B. Yu, MD**
Chief Resident
Department of Therapeutic
    Radiology
Yale-New Haven Hospital
New Haven, Connecticut
*Chapter 2: Radiation Therapy for
    Brain Metastases*
*Chapter 3: Prognosis of Patients
    with Brain Metastases Who
    Undergo Radiation Therapy*

# Brain Metastasis

# 1

# Neurologic Manifestations of Brain Metastases
## Recognition, Evolution, and Management

Jessica Kraker
Jaishri Blakeley

Neurologic disease is a common problem in patients with systemic cancers. Metastatic disease to the central nervous system (CNS), treatment related neurologic toxicities, or paraneoplastic syndromes can all cause neurologic signs and symptoms. Twenty to forty percent of all patients with systemic malignancies develop brain metastases at some time in the disease course (1–3). In addition, the incidence and prevalence of brain metastases are increasing, possibly due to improved long-term control of systemic disease and increased recognition of the disease (3,4). Hence, brain metastases are a major source of disability, morbidity, and mortality in cancer patients.

Brain metastases may present with a wide variety of signs and symptoms, ranging from an incidental finding on imaging to mental status changes, seizures, or focal neurological deficits such as weakness or aphasia. Early identification and management of these tumors may improve function and possibly survival. Hence, a high index of suspicion for brain metastases is required. This chapter presents the most common neurologic signs and symptoms of brain metastases, the diagnostic procedures currently available, and a discussion about initial management when a brain metastasis is diagnosed.

## Tumor Types and Patterns of CNS Metastases

The most common route of spread of cancer cells from the periphery to the CNS is hematogenous, with cancer entering either from the internal carotid or vertebrobasilar arteries or from the Baton venous plexus along the spinal cord.

1

Metastatic cells preferentially localize at the junction of the brain gray and white matter and in vascular "border zones" between two major vascular supplies (Figure 1.1). This is likely due to the decreasing caliber of the blood vessels in these areas limiting further progression of the cells. As the greatest volume of blood supply flows to the cortex, this is the most common site for brain metastases (80 percent), followed by the cerebellum (15 percent), and brainstem (5 percent) (2,5). However, patients with both solid and hematologic malignancies may also have diffuse infiltration of the leptomeninges. The most common cancers to cause leptomeningeal disease, both in children and adults, are the acute leukemias and lymphomas. Solid tumors also cause leptomeningeal disease, however, this often occurs only after progression of an intraparenchymal metastasis (6).

The most common solid tumors associated with brain metastases are lung, breast, and gastrointestinal cancers (1). This is largely because these are the most common cancers in the population overall. Other tumors, such as melanoma, renal cell carcinoma, and choriocarcinoma, are less common but have a high propensity to metastasize to the brain (1,5). Melanoma, renal cell carcinoma, choriocarcinoma, and thyroid carcinomas are also the most common tumor types to present with intracranial hemorrhage, whereas metastases from GI cancers are more likely to have mucoid components or fluid-filled cysts.

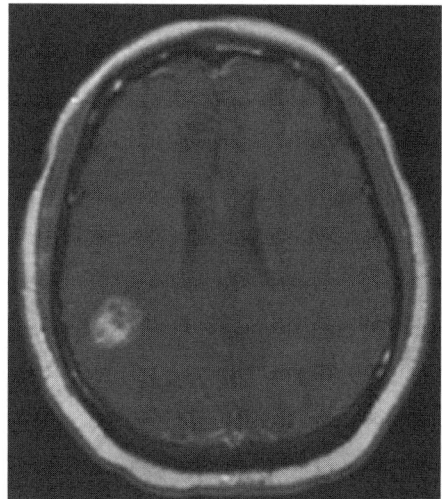

FIGURE 1.1    MRI image of brain, T1w axial image demonstrating a contrast enhancing lesion at the gray-white junction in the cortex from a patient with widely metastatic breast cancer and new onset headache.

## Symptoms of Brain Metastases

The area of brain involved by the metastasis and associated edema will dictate the symptoms the patient experiences. Signs and symptoms can be categorized into those that are localizable (associated neuroanatomically with specific findings) and those that are general. General symptoms (headache, somnolence, confusion, nausea) may be caused by elevated intracranial pressure or may be independent of structural neurologic disease. General symptoms are both the most common and the most difficult to approach clinically as they can represent a spectrum of disease from no neurologic disease to impending herniation. The most common general neurologic manifestations of brain metastases are discussed below. Focal manifestations are discussed in the next section.

### Headache

Headache is one of the most common presenting complaints of the general population. In fact, as many as 12 to 16 percent of otherwise healthy people meet the criteria for migraine (7). Headaches are also a common side effect of many chemotherapies. Common primary headaches (such as tension or migraine headaches) can be exacerbated by the situations cancer patients regularly experience and are a common complaint among patients with cancer that does not always require extensive work up.

However, headache is also a common presenting symptom for brain metastasis. Roughly 32 to 54 percent of patients with a systemic malignancy who present with new onset headache or a change in baseline headache are found to have a brain metastasis (8,9). Similarly, 48 to 80 percent of patients with a known diagnosis of primary or metastatic brain tumors complain of headaches (8,10).

There are no specific features of headache that predict the presence of a brain metastasis; in fact, the "classic" headache features thought to correspond to brain tumors (severe headache, worse in the morning, associated with nausea and vomiting) were found in only in 9 of 111 patients (8 percent) with brain tumors (10). In contrast, 71 percent of patients with known brain tumors have headaches that are most consistent with common tension headaches (dull pain, nonpositional). Hence, a high index of suspicion is required for patients with a history of cancer presenting with new or worsening headaches. The severity and rapidity of the headache, the associated symptoms, and physical exam findings can help determine the urgency of the evaluation.

A detailed history may help determine whether the patient is suffering from a primary headache syndrome (such as tension, migraine, or cluster headache) or a secondary headache (related to a space-occupying lesion). Headaches that are new, severe, and reach peak intensity rapidly are likely to be secondary. A brief memory device to assess if a headache needs emergent attention is "First, Worst, and Cursed" (Table 1.1). If it is the first headache a patient has ever experienced and it is unremitting or escalating, imaging with a computed tomography (CT) of the head or magnetic resonance imaging (MRI) of the brain is needed urgently.

If the patient reports it is the "worst" headache he or she has ever experienced, an urgent evaluation is recommended both for diagnosis of secondary causes such as tumor, bleed, or infection, as well as for pain management. Headaches that are "cursed" are associated with new focal neurological deficits and are almost always the result of a structural lesion or elevated intracranial pressure (ICP). Patients with these headaches require emergent clinical evaluation including neuroimaging with either a noncontrast head CT or a contrast enhanced MRI brain. The differential diagnosis in these cases includes new metastasis, intracranial hemorrhage, infection, or hydrocephalus.

Headaches associated with symptoms such as blurred vision or obscured vision (due to pressure on the optic nerve), diplopia (often due to pressure on the trochanter nerve), confusion, or vomiting, or a headache that is worse upon waking, with coughing or the valsalva maneuver, may indicate increased ICP. A fundoscopic examination should be performed to evaluate for papilledema (optic disc swelling), which confirms elevated ICP. A lumbar puncture (LP) can confirm elevated ICP by measuring the opening pressure and also assist in the diagnostic work-up for etiologies such as infection, subarachnoid hemorrhage, or leptomeningeal disease. It is important to recall that in all cases of suspected elevated ICP, neuroimaging is required prior to LP to ensure there is no significant mass effect that could result in herniation when cerebrospinal fluid (CSF) is drained. Only after a full work-up is negative, should a patient with cancer and a new, severe headache with focal neurologic deficits be considered to have a primary headache syndrome such as migraine.

If there is a prior history of headaches, it is important to delineate the pattern of head pain a patient usually experiences (quality, frequency, severity) and any new changes in that pattern. Chronic headache syndromes can be exacer-

TABLE 1.1  Rapid Evaluation of Headaches—Triage Questions and Responses Suggestive of a Secondary Headache

| QUESTIONS | RESPONSES THAT RAISE CONCERN |
| --- | --- |
| When did the headache begin? | New headaches within the last 4–10 weeks |
| What is the quality and severity of your pain? | Severe |
| Was the pain at its worst from the start or has it built steadily over time? | Acute, maximal onset pain. Suggests a mass lesion or bleed. Classic terms are "thunderclap" or "worst headache of my life." |
| Do you get headaches regularly? If so, is this headache different from the headaches you have experienced in the past? | New or newly changed headache. |
| Are there any associated symptoms such as fever, nausea, vomiting, visual changes, confusion, trouble speaking, numbness, tingling, or weakness? | Focal neurologic deficits, change in mental status or fever are emergencies. Nausea and vomiting may be associated with primary headache syndrome, but need further evaluation with neuroimaging. |
| Are there any provoking or alleviating factors? Does the headache change with position, coughing, Valsalva maneuvers? | Headaches that are worse when supine (or present upon waking, but improve with sitting up), coughing or Valsalva are suggestive of elevated intracranial pressure. |

bated by factors such as medications, stress, and sleep disruption. Hence, it is not uncommon for patients with known underlying chronic headaches to have more frequent headaches during cancer therapy. More aggressive management of an underlying headache syndrome may be warranted in such instances. Neuroimaging is warranted whenever there is a new quality or severity of pain or new associated neurologic symptoms.

The urgency of evaluation for patients complaining of headache also depends on the situation in which the headache arises. A fever accompanying new onset severe headache raises concern for meningitis requiring emergent evaluation. Acute onset of headache after retching or intense exercise suggests a dissection or possible intracranial hemorrhage. Headache that reaches maximal intensity rapidly with or without focal neurologic deficits is also suggestive of a hemorrhage.

A common cause of intracranial bleed in all patients is hypertension. The most common locations for hypertensive bleeds are the brainstem, thalamus, and cerebellum (11). These patients require emergent evaluation for blood pressure and acute neurologic disease management. Patients with underlying malignancy are also at risk for dyscoagulation, which increases the risk of intracranial bleed or thrombosis. Finally, brain metastases may present as hemorrhagic lesions. This is particularly true with melanoma, renal cell carcinoma, thyroid cancer, and choriocarcinoma, but can occur with any tumor. For this reason, all patients with known systemic malignancy that present with an acute brain hemorrhage should undergo follow-up brain MRI three months after presentation to evaluate for an underlying mass regardless of what the initial etiology for the hemorrhage is thought to be.

## Seizure

Seizures are another common presentation of metastatic disease, with 14 to 51 percent of patients with both primary and metastatic brain tumors presenting with seizures (12,13). A seizure is a paroxysmal, transient defect in neurological functioning resulting from excessive aberrant electrical discharge from neurons of the cerebral cortex. The actual clinical presentation of the electrical discharges has a great deal of variability, including episodic confusion, brief starring episodes, feelings of fear or déjà vu, and the most dramatic: a generalized tonic-clonic seizure characterized by loss of consciousness and diffuse shaking and stiffening.

Seizure types can be grouped into two main categories: partial and generalized. With partial seizures, focal areas of the brain are involved and the manifestations are localized to one limb or area. Generalized seizures are events that begin simultaneously in both hemispheres of the brain. Partial seizures are more common than generalized seizures and can be further classified as simple or complex seizures. A simple seizure involves shaking of one region of the body. A seizure becomes "complex" whenever consciousness is altered in any way. A common complex partial seizure is an aura of some form (odd smell, taste, or sensation) followed by shaking of one side accompanied by unresponsiveness. Patterns of seizure presentation may help localize a seizure to a particular region of the brain, and common patterns are described in Table 1.6.

A partial seizure also has the potential to progress from focal to generalized if spontaneous discharges spread to involve the whole brain. This is called a secondary generalized seizure. After such an event, there may be a period of confusion and decreased alertness called a post-ictal state. Although in some cases there can be a prolonged post-ictal state, altered mental status lasting beyond half an hour after a seizure has subsided should prompt further evaluation for subclinical seizures or another underlying process. Finally, patients may experience weakness of one side of the body that can mimic a stroke. This is known as Todd's paralysis, and the weakness can persist for several hours. Again, deficits that persist beyond hours or a day should be further evaluated with neuroimaging.

Patients with known systemic cancer who present with a new onset seizure require neuroimaging with brain MRI. If a metastasis is identified, chronic anticonvulsant therapy is required. There are numerous antiepileptic drugs, each with indications for use in specific seizure types. Commonly used antiepileptic medications include phenytoin, carbamazepine, leviteracetam, lamotrigine, and gabapentin. All agents have similar efficacy and should be chosen based on their potential side effects and drug interactions. Side effects to be kept in mind when prescribing an antiepileptic drug for patients with brain cancer include cognitive impairment, myelosupression, and possible drug-drug interactions with chemotherapeutic agents. Newer generation agents such as leviteracetam, lamotrigine, and gabapentin are generally preferable for this patient population.

There is currently no evidence to support treating patients with brain metastasis with prophylactic anticonvulsants if they have never had a seizure (12). If a patient with systemic cancer presents with a seizure but no brain metastasis or leptomeningeal disease can be identified, evaluation for other precipitating causes (infection, medication effect, metabolic derangement) is warranted. Chronic antiseizure management is likely not required if an etiology can be identified and reversed. If an underlying etiology is not identified and the value of chronic antiseizure medication in unclear, an electroencephalogram (EEG) can help identify a focal area of irritation that would suggest a need for chronic antiseizure medication.

## Fatigue

Fatigue is one of the most pervasive complaints among patients with cancer (14,15). It is often multifactorial and related to the underlying malignancy as well as the required therapies, including surgery, radiation, and chemotherapy (16). Generalized fatigue is rarely the result of a neurologic syndrome. However, patients with profound fatigue resulting in excessive sleep or difficulty in waking or maintaining arousal should be evaluated for a neurologic process. Disease of bilateral frontal lobes, bilateral thalamic nuclei, the brain stem or the leptomeninges, or elevated ICP from any cause, can all result in significantly decreased attention and drowsiness. Patients presenting with profoundly decreased alertness should undergo neuroimaging early in the evaluation. If leptomeningeal disease is suspected, an LP is required.

## Altered Mental Status

Cognitive dysfunction is a common complaint among patients with cancer and can present in many forms, from subtle memory dysfunction and difficulty concentrating to overt disorientation, hallucinations, or lethargy. Acute changes in mental status are a common cause for hospital admission for all cancer patients, but they do not always reflect brain metastases (17). In fact, in the majority of cancer patients with acute mental status changes, multiple potential contributing etiologies were identified independent of brain metastases. That said, in one series, 25 percent of patients with systemic malignancy and new cognitive changes were found to have brain metastases (18). Hence, although brain metastases should be considered when evaluating any acute change in mental status in patients with known malignancy, a full evaluation for all causes of acute change in mental status is required.

Delirium is characterized by acute to subacute onset of confusion with fluctuating mental status. Common causes of delirium include infection, hemorrhage or stroke, hypoxia, metabolic changes (most commonly hypo- or hyperglycemia or hyponatremia), new or changed medications, or toxins. It is important to recognize delirium early because although delirium can be fatal, if caught early and an etiology is identified, it can be fully reversed (19). Patients with cancer are at risk for many of the causes of delirium, and basic investigation for factors contributing to delirium should be pursued. However, simultaneous evaluation for brain metastases is warranted. Symptom reversal occurred in up to two-thirds of patients who presented with delirium, were found to have brain metastases, and were treated with glucocorticoids (18). Finally, intermittent disorientation or transient changes in consciousness that appear to be similar to delirium may in fact be due to subclinical seizures. If this is suspected in a patient with a history of cancer, both neuroimaging and an EEG are required.

More subtle and chronic cognitive changes can be seen during or after radiation therapy or chemotherapy. There is increasing recognition of diffuse cognitive dysfunction associated with multiple chemotherapies coined "chemo brain" in the popular press. This is characterized by a wide array of neurocognitive difficulties, such as impaired concentration, short-term memory loss, and impaired executive function (20). The problem was first recognized in breast cancer patients who were found to have a 25 to 40 percent frequency of cognitive dysfunction based on formal neuropsychiatric testing and is increasingly recognized among survivors of other solid tumors (20–22).

In summary, mild to moderate cognitive dysfunction is common in cancer patients in the absence of cancer-related CNS disease. If the cognitive findings are subtle and gradual, extensive neurologic work-up is likely not required. Neuropsychiatric testing may be helpful to guide cognitive and behavioral therapies but are not necessary urgently. However, acute changes in cognition or alertness are always worrisome and work-up of causes of delirium, including neuroimaging to detect brain metastases should be pursued.

## Focal Neurologic Deficits: Localizing the Disease

The brain is divided into distinct areas that control different aspects of cognitive and physical function (Figure 1.2). Familiarity with the anatomy of the CNS can help identify deficits (allowing recognition of the possibility of a metastasis) and localize lesions prior to imaging. After imaging, this can help the clinician advise patients about potential functional limitations.

Deficits from brain metastases can be caused by multiple mechanisms. The tumor may invade brain parenchyma and destroy nervous system tissue. The tumor or tumor-related edema may exert pressure on the surrounding tissue. Brain tumors may also cause vascular compromise resulting in hemorrhagic or ischemic stroke, either by co-opting normal blood vessels or through tumor angiogenesis creating unstable new vessels (23). As there are many mechanisms by which brain metastases can cause neurologic deficits, the time course for symptom presentation can be highly variable. Symptoms arising from tumor compression or edema tend to occur subacutely, whereas vascular events are acute.

The central nervous system contains the cerebral cortex, the diencephalon (thalamus, hypothalamus), the limbic system, the brainstem (midbrain, pons, medulla), the cerebellum, and the spinal cord. The cerebral cortex is divided down the middle into a left and right hemisphere. Each hemisphere is divided into four lobes: the frontal, parietal, occipital, and temporal lobes (Figure 1.2). Each region has a unique set of primary functions and there is lateral dominance for many functions.

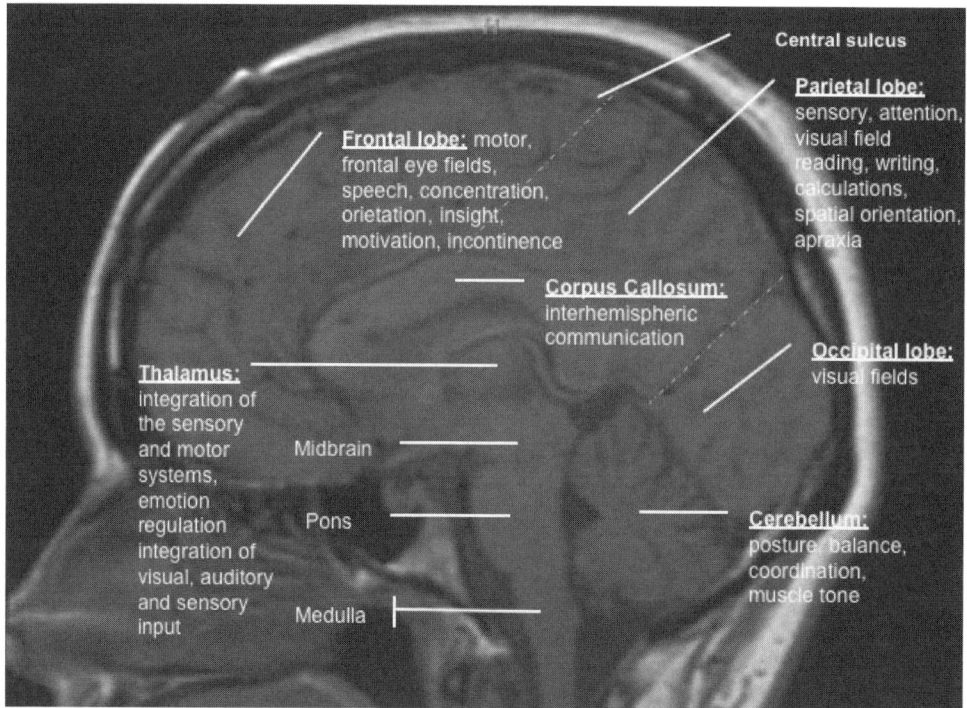

**Central sulcus**

**Parietal lobe:** sensory, attention, visual field reading, writing, calculations, spatial orientation, apraxia

**Frontal lobe:** motor, frontal eye fields, speech, concentration, orietation, insight, motivation, incontinence

**Corpus Callosum:** interhemispheric communication

**Occipital lobe:** visual fields

**Thalamus:** integration of the sensory and motor systems, emotion regulation integration of visual, auditory and sensory input

Midbrain

Pons

Medulla

**Cerebellum:** posture, balance, coordination, muscle tone

FIGURE 1.2    Sagittal view of the brain on T1w MRI with critical anatomic regions and their functions highlighted.

## Frontal Lobe

The frontal lobe has multiple important functions, including motor function, language, attention, motivation, executive functioning, judgment, planning, and problem solving (Table 1.2) (24). Motor weakness is one of the most common focal signs in patients with brain metastases (3). Focal weakness can originate from multiple sources, including muscle, peripheral nerve, or spinal cord. Patterns of signs and symptoms help localize the source of weakness. Peripheral nervous system lesions (root, nerve, or muscle) have distinct features from those found in CNS lesions (Table 1.3). Lesions of the spinal cord present with CNS patterns of weakness, however, they are often associated with back pain, a sensory level or bowel or bladder dysfunction. In contrast, lesions in the CNS that cause weakness will commonly involve an entire limb, be accompanied by sensory loss in the same distribution as the weakness, may be associated with other cortical functions such as speech difficulty, and are not associated with pain.

The primary motor cortex is located on the precentral gyrus, just in front of the central sulcus (Figure 1.2). Most of the cortical spinal tract originates

TABLE 1.2  The Divisions of the Central Nervous System and Their Major Roles

| DIVISION OF CENTRAL NERVOUS SYSTEM | MAJOR FUNCTIONS |
| --- | --- |
| Frontal Lobes | Forethought and planning, executive functions, personality, premotor cortex, motor cortex |
| Parietal Lobes | Somatosensory cortex, perception, integrating input to construct spatial coordinate system for world around us. Visual pathways. |
| Temporal Lobes | Memory, auditory receptive area, language. Visual pathways. |
| Occipital Lobes | Visual reception and interpretation |
| Limbic System | Includes amygdala, hypothalamus, hippocampus: integration of memory, emotions, homeostasis |
| Cerebellum | Coordination, balance, tone |
| Brain Stem | Cranial nerves, pathway to spinal cord, cardiac and respiratory function |
| Spinal Cord | Relays motor information to periphery, and sensory information to CNS |

here. The cortical fibers cross at the level of the midbrain in the brainstem, so that fibers from the left motor cortex supply muscles on the right side of the body. The motor cortex is further arranged in a representation of the body known as the homunculus (Figure 1.3). In this internal map of the body, the leg is represented over the medial aspect of the brain, the arm and hand extend around to the lateral side of the brain, with the face represented most inferiorly and laterally. This representation allows further localization of exam findings. For example, left hand weakness is traceable to the right superior frontal lobe.

The prefrontal cortex is the large anterior portion of the frontal lobe and holds the orbitofrontal, ventromedial, dorsolateral prefrontal, and the cingulate cortex (24). Together these regions of the frontal lobe are responsible for higher order cognitive function such as decision making, motor planning,

TABLE 1.3  Distinguishing Central from Peripheral Weakness

| SIGNS | CENTRAL NERVOUS SYSTEM | PERIPHERAL NERVOUS SYSTEM |
| --- | --- | --- |
| Weakness | Yes | Yes |
| Atrophy | Yes | Yes |
| Fasciculations | No | Yes |
| Reflexes | Increased | Decreased |

FIGURE 1.3   Motor and sensory homunculus demonstrating the representation of peripheral function along the motor and sensory cortex. The motor cortex is along the precentral gyrus in the frontal lobe and the sensory cortex is on the postcentral gyrus in the parietal lobe. Differential representation is given to hand, face, and mouth, reflecting critical functions instead of functions critical to our species.

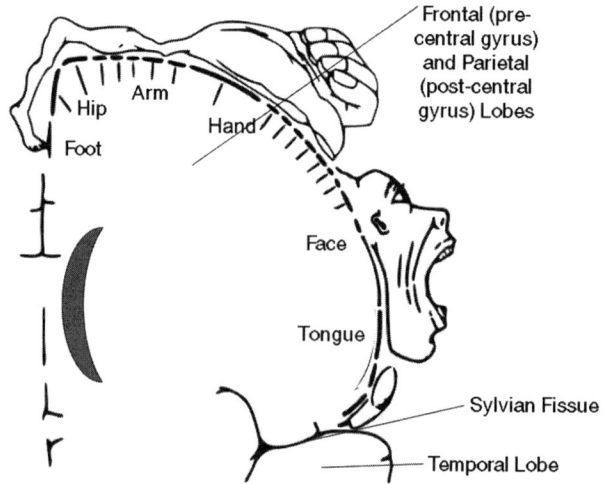

abstract thinking, risk assessment, integration of information and socialization, emotional regulation, and attention. Hence, damage to the prefrontal cortex may cause a broad range of behavioral and cognitive deficits, including personality changes, erratic behavior, and depression. Bilateral involvement of the frontal lobes can lead to severely decreased attention and alertness and, in extreme cases, coma.

Finally, the frontal lobe holds critical areas for language production, including Broca's area (dominant inferior frontal lobe) that is responsible for speech production. Tumors in the left inferior frontal lobe often present with inability to produce speech with preserved comprehension. Other critical functions mediated by the frontal lobe are voluntary eye movements for tracking controlled by the frontal eye fields.

## Parietal Lobe

The parietal lobes are located behind the frontal lobe posterior to the central sulcus and extend to the occipital lobe (Figure 1.2) and have four main functions: sensation, perception, vision, and spatial and visual integration. The somatosensory cortex is organized along a homunculus like the motor cortex (Figure 1.3). The ascending sensory pathways that terminate in the somatosensory cortex are also crossed. Hence, a lesion in the left parietal lobe will be associated with abnormal sensation on the right. The parietal lobes also control higher order sensory processing, such as the ability to discriminate between two points of stimulation, the ability to determine what an object is by touch, or to detect a number or letter traced on the hand. Deficits in these skills are termed astereognosia and agraphasthesia, respectively.

There are distinct functions in the two sides of the parietal lobe. Injuries to the dominant parietal lobe (often the left parietal lobe in a right-handed person) can result in right-left confusion, inability to recognize fingers, and an inability to read, write, or do calculations. This collection of deficits is termed "Gerstman's Syndrome." Injuries to the nondominant parietal lobe (often the right parietal lobe) can result in neglect of the contralateral world to the extent that patients may not recognize their own body parts or objects on their left despite fully functional vision. Other syndromes of the nondominant parietal lobe are lack of awareness of deficits or denial of illness (anosognosia).

Parietal lobe lesions can also cause apraxia—an inability to perform a complex collection of movements necessary to complete a specific task (such as brushing teeth or hammering a nail). This inability to complete a motor task can occur even though motor and sensory function are normal.

Finally, the optic radiations travel through the parietal lobe on their way from the optic chiasm to the occipital lobe. Fibers from the contralateral, inferior visual fields travel through the parietal lobe. Unilateral lesions in the parietal lobe may cause contralateral inferior visual field loss called an inferior quadrantanopsia. In addition, bilateral parietal lobe lesions can cause a visual integration syndrome called "Balint's Syndrome" in which patients cannot integrate the multiple components in their view into a unified scene and cannot guide their eye movements.

In summary, patients that present with odd symptoms centered around an inability to sense or integrate external stimuli or to coordinate task-based actions, despite intact motor function, should be evaluated for parietal lobe lesions.

## Temporal Lobe

The temporal lobes are located below the frontal and parietal lobes. The dominant temporal lobe houses several critical areas, including Wernicke's area, the hippocampus, and the auditory cortex. Wernicke's area is involved in language comprehension. Injury here results in a receptive aphasia (patients cannot comprehend speech but can produce fluent speech). The nondominant lobe contributes to recognition of changes in tone of voice and music, and damage here results in impaired ability to recognize tone of speech. Given the role the temporal lobes play in interpretation of auditory stimuli, it is not surprising that the primary auditory cortex is just anterior to Wernicke's area. Bilateral lesions of the medial superior temporal gyrus can therefore result in cortical deafness, however, unilateral injury results in only mild hearing loss.

The temporal lobes also house the hippocampus and amygdala. The hippocampus is the region responsible for consolidation of new memories. The amygdala is a major nucleus in the limbic cortex and contributes to regulation of emotion and to new learning. These structures are redundant to the extent that damage to both sides is required to cause a symptomatic deficit. Damage to bilateral hippocampi results in the inability to store new memories. Damage to bilateral amygdala results in apathy and difficulty assessing others' emotional states (25). If the anterior portions of bilateral temporal lobes (including both the amygdala and hippocampi) are injured, a syndrome of psychic blindness, docility, and disinhibition, termed Kluver-Bucy syndrome, may result (26). Finally, the inferior tracts of the optic radiations traveling from the chiasm to the occipital lobe are in the temporal lobe. These fibers are responsible for the superior, contralateral visual fields, and injury causes a superior quadrantanopsia (opposite from what occurs with a parietal lobe lesion).

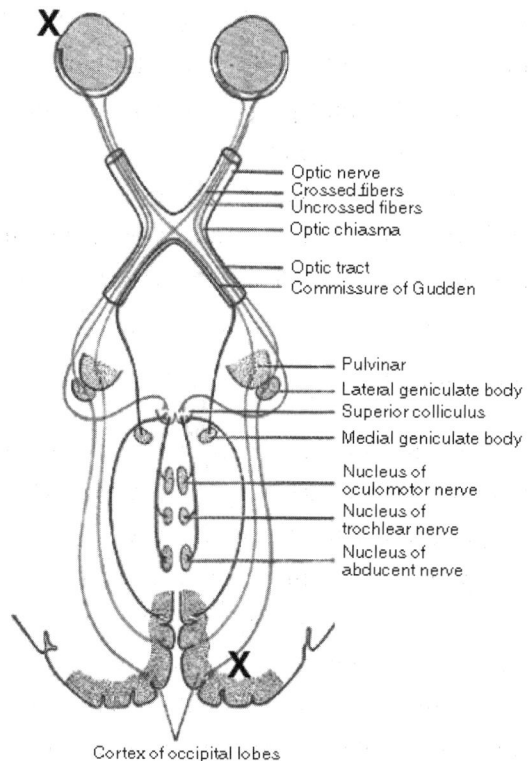

X

Optic nerve
Crossed fibers
Uncrossed fibers
Optic chiasma

Optic tract
Commissure of Gudden

Pulvinar
Lateral geniculate body
Superior colliculus
Medial geniculate body

Nucleus of
oculomotor nerve
Nucleus of
trochlear nerve
Nucleus of
abducent nerve

X

Cortex of occipital lobes

FIGURE 1.4 Schematic of the optic pathways adapted from 20th U.S. edition of *Gray's Anatomy of the Human Body*.

## Occipital Lobe

The occipital lobes hold the visual cortex. The information is laid out on the occipital lobe in reverse of the information received by the retina. For example, the image projected onto the inferior visual field will be represented in the superior occipital lobe (Figure 1.4). Incoming visual information follows a pathway from the retina to the optic nerves that travel through the temporal lobes (superior field) and parietal lobes (inferior field) to the occipital lobe. The information from the lateral aspect of each retina remains ipsilateral, whereas information from the nasal aspect of the retina crosses at the optic chiasm to the contralateral side. Lesions of the occipital lobe may cause hemianopsia (if unilateral) or cortical blindness (if bilateral). Lesions of the occipital lobe may also cause visual hallucinations as can be seen in the Charles Bonnet syndrome characterized by isolated complex visual hallucinations (27).

## Deep Nuclei and Brainstem

The diencephalon is a primitive part of the brain that contains the thalamus and hypothalamus. The thalamus is the key relay station of the brain, sending information from the cortex to the periphery and vice versa. It is arranged like a miniature cerebral cortex, with multiple named nuclei, each with a specific responsibility. Hence, thalamic lesions may result in cognitive, motor, sensory, coordination, behavioral, visual, or auditory deficits (28). The most common manifestations of thalamic lesions are cognitive and behavior disorders (28,29). However, there can be isolated motor or sensory dysfunction of an entire side (hemiparesis, hemisensory loss) contralateral to a thalamic lesion or to a lesion of the internal capsule (30). Alternatively, large lesions of the thalamus may be relatively asymptomatic, especially if they are infiltrative.

The hypothalamus is just below the thalamus. It is a regulatory center connecting the pituitary gland and the brain to regulate hormonal and endocrine systems. This nucleus is rarely involved directly by metastatic disease to the brain, however, the therapies that are used to treat brain cancer can effect hypothalamic-pituitary function and result in hypothyroidism, adrenal insufficiency, or diabetes insipidus (31). There are also rare cases of metastases to the pituitary gland. In these instances, symptoms often include both hypothalamic-pituitary endocrine dysfunction as well as visual abnormalities (32,33). In cancer patients with vague systemic complaints, screening endocrinologic studies are likely sufficient to detect whether hypothalamic-pituitary damage has occurred as a result of cancer therapies. However, in cancer patients with new visual abnormalities and endrocrinologic complaints, neuroimaging is required to assess for metastatic involvement of the pituitary complex.

The brain stem contains the midbrain, pons, and medulla, and connects the brain to the spinal cord. It is the control center of the CNS and holds all of the tracts that carry information between the brain and spinal cord. The motor tracks cross at the level of the medulla so lesions above the medulla result in contralateral weakness and lesions below the medulla result in ipsilateral weakness. The brainstem also houses the nuclei of the cranial nerves, which control the motor output and sensation of the eyes, face, and oropharynx (Table 1.4). The close proximity of the motor tracks traveling through the brainstem and the cranial nerve nuclei results in the most salient localizing feature of brain-stem lesions: "crossed findings". This is defined as ipsilateral cranial nerve deficits (facial weakness, occulomotor weakness, loss of facial sensation, etc.) with contralateral body weakness and occurs anywhere in the brain stem above the mid-lower medulla.

TABLE 1.4 Cranial Nerve Functions

| CRANIAL NERVES | FUNCTION |
| --- | --- |
| CN I Olfactory nerve | Sense of smell |
| CN II Optic nerve | Visual information |
| CN III Oculomotor nerve | Pupil constriction, controls eye movements with superior, inferior and medial rectus muscles |
| CN IV Trochlear nerve | Controls moving eye up via inferior oblique |
| CN V Trigeminal nerve | Has three branches, V1–V3, that control face sensation, and the sensory aspect of the corneal reflex, Masseter muscle |
| CN VI Abducens nerve | Abducts the eye via lateral rectus muscle |
| CN VII Facial nerve | Taste anterior 2/3 of the tongue, sensation of outer ear, face muscles, stapedius |
| CN VIII Vestibular-cochlear nerve | Hearing, equilibrium |
| CN XI Glossopharyngeal | External ear sensation, taste on posterior 1/3 of tongue, pharynx, carotid body, parotid gland, sensory part of gag reflex |
| CN X Vagus nerve | Elevates palate, swallowing |
| CN XI Accessory nerve | Controls head turning via sternocleidomastoids and shoulder shrug via trapezious muscles. |
| CN XII Hypoglossal nerve | Tongue muscles |

## Cerebellum

The cerebellum is dorsal to the brain stem and is divided into a right and left hemisphere. It has three main functions: coordinating motor movement, contributing to maintaining balance, and maintaining muscle tone. The cerebellar peduncles communicate between the cerebellum and the brain stem, and lesions in these areas will manifest similarly to cerebellar lesions. Lesions in the cerebellum often result in ipsilateral dysmetria and ataxia. This is unique from the rest of the cerebral cortex organization.

## Leptomeningeal Disease

The leptomeninges is the protective layering of the CNS and comprises two layers: the arachnoid and the pia mater. Cancer spread to the leptomeninges occurs in 5 to 10 percent of patients with solid tumors and up to 35 percent of patients with leukemia and lymphomas (34). Of the solid tumors, breast and lung tumors are most likely to metastasize to the leptomeninges, followed by melanoma and gastrointestinal cancers (35). The incidence of breast and lung metastasis to the leptomeninges appears to be increasing, possibly due to improved systemic control of disease and improved neuroimaging (35). The solid tumors of the head and neck, thyroid, prostate, and bladder are overall unlikely to seed the leptomeninges (36).

Metastatic cancer cells reach the meninges in one of four manners: hematogenous spread, direct extension from preexisting tumor in brain parenchyma, epidural or ventricular space along perineural or perivascular lymphatics, or iatrogenic spread during procedures (6,35). Once the tumor cells breach the meninges, they circulate through the CSF and are carried to other parts of the neuraxis, settling in gravity dependent areas.

The clinical manifestations of leptomeningeal disease take many forms, depending on which portion of the neuraxis is affected. One of the most common presentations is multiple cranial nerve dysfunction. Diplopia with occuloparesis is a common cranial nerve (CN) manifestation. Additional common cranial nerve deficits with leptomeningeal disease are facial hemiparesis, difficulty swallowing, and decreased hearing. Any new cranial nerve palsy in a patient with known cancer warrants evaluation for leptomeningeal disease.

Up to 60 percent of patients with leptomeningeal carcinomatosis will have radicular nerve symptoms (distal weakness, neuropathic back pain) related to involvement of the nerve roots. This high frequency may be due to the tendency of tumor cells to settle at the dependent portion of the neuraxis, often along the cauda equina and sacral nerve roots (35).

Another common manifestation is altered mental status with or without headache (36). This presentation suggests cancer cells have coated the leptomeninges, resulting in a communicating hydrocephalus with associated elevated ICP. Patients may also experience nausea and vomiting, cognitive changes, and occasionally seizures due to the involvement of the meninges.

If leptomeningeal carcinomatosis is suspected, a brain and spine MRI with contrast followed by an LP for opening pressure (measured with the patient in a lateral decubitus position), cell count, protein level, glucose level, and cytology should be pursued. The presence of malignant cells within the CSF is the defining feature of leptomeningeal disease. CSF findings consistent with leptomeningeal involvement also include elevated opening pressure, significantly elevated protein, and possibly elevated cell count and decreased glucose (Table 1.5). Tumors with predilection both for hemorrhage and leptomeningeal involvement such as melanoma, thyroid carcinoma, chorionic carcinoma, and renal cell carcinoma may also have elevated red blood cell counts or xanthochromic CSF.

Roughly 47 to 90 percent of patients with leptomeningeal involvement from a metastatic tumor will have positive cytology (although this may require repeat sampling), and nearly 100 percent will have abnormal CSF studies (36–40). Overall, there is an 84 percent sensitivity for recovering cells in clinically suspected leptomeningeal disease after two or more samplings (39). These findings are the basis for the recommendation that two to three large volume (greater than 20mL) lumbar punctures be done to assess for the malignant cells in CSF in patients with suspected leptomeningeal metastases. The specificity of CSF studies for leptomeningeal disease is 100 percent, however, the sensitivity

TABLE 1.5 Summary of Findings in Leptomeningeal Disease

| Opening Pressure | 60–550 MM $H_2O$ |
|---|---|
| Protein | 24–2400 mg/100ml |
| Cell Count | 0–1800cells/mm$^3$<br>Lymphocytic & mononuclear predominance |
| Glucose | 0–225 mg/100ml |
| Positive Cytology | Positive 45–90% of cases<br>Commonly requires 2–3 samples |

is much lower and again, dependent to some extent on the number of lumbar punctures performed. In contrast, MRI has a sensitivity of 76 percent and a specificity of 77 percent (41). A positive result on either MRI or CSF is sufficient for diagnosing leptomeningeal carcinomatosis in patients with the appropriate clinical symptoms. However, in many cases both studies are needed. Some important operational points are 1) the LP should be done after an MRI to avoid artifactual enhancement of the dura secondary to pressure changes after CSF drainage, and 2) CSF studies are more likely to be positive if drawn from the lumbar space rather than a shunt or ventricular catheter.

## Diagnosis of Brain Metastasis

Neuroimaging is the most important diagnostic modality for CNS metastases. This includes computed tomography (CT scan) of the head and brain MRI. Although MRI is the gold standard for diagnosing CNS metastatic disease, CT scans are rapid and widely available (42–44). Hence, if a patient needs acute evaluation, a CT head scan should be obtained as the preliminary test to assess for intracranial hemorrhage, significant mass effect, or hydrocephalus. If a bleed is suspected, contrast should not be given. In the absence of exogenous contrast, most metastatic lesions will be isodense (appearing the same density) to the surrounding brain parenchyma on head CT and may be hard to identify. Areas of asymmetry may be apparent, but exogenous contrast (iodinated for CT, gadolinium for MRI) will ultimately be needed for anatomical definition.

As soon as is feasible, a brain MRI with contrast should be obtained. An MRI has much more sensitivity than a CT for identifying lesions in the posterior fossa, assessing for leptomeningeal or ependymal involvement, detecting small parenchymal lesions, and assessing the extent of edema. General MRI features are distinct mass lesions at the gray-white junction that have heterogenous contrast enhancement (possibly ring enhancing) with significant associated edema (T2w hyperintensity). Specific MRI features depend to some extent on the primary tumor. For example, melanoma can be both hypointense on T2w images and hyperintense of T1w images, which is atypical for all other tumors and is due to the melanin content (45).

Although a standard MRI has excellent anatomical detail, it has limited specificity. This is significant when trying to assess the etiology of a single lesion identified on an MRI as well as when trying to assess the response of tumor to therapy. In as many as 11 percent of patients with systemic cancer, an

TABLE 1.6 Localization of Seizure Features

| CLINICAL FEATURE | LOCALIZATION |
|---|---|
| Complex visual hallucinations | Posterior temporal or occipital lobes |
| Olfactory hallucinations | Inferior and medial temporal lobe |
| Automatisms, such as picking at clothes repeatedly | Frontal or temporal lobes |
| Focal Motor | Prerolandic gyrus (frontal lobes) |
| Head turning, eye turning, with arm movements | Supplementary motor cortex |
| Auditory hallucination | Heschl's gyri |
| Affective states such as fear, déjà vu, depersonalization | Temporal lobe |

new, single brain lesion is not due to metastasis but rather to a primary brain tumor or infection (46). As patients receive more and more therapy for brain cancer, it is also becoming more difficult to assess which MRI changes are due to treatment effect and which are related to progressive tumors (47). Alternative imaging modalities such as FDG PET, MR spectroscopy, diffusion tensor imaging, and cerebral blood volume measures are being applied to try to distinguish the various types of tumors and to differentiate tumors from treatment-related injuries (48–51). While this research is promising, there are no validated studies to date.

If a lesion is identified on an MRI and there is a question of whether it represents metastasis, staging of the systemic cancer can be helpful. If there is no other sign of systemic disease, the likelihood of an isolated brain metastasis is reduced and a biopsy is indicated to determine the etiology. Alternatively, if there is evidence of widely metastatic disease, a contemporous lesion on brain MRI is likely to represent metastasis.

In summary, when there is any suspicion of brain metastasis, brain MRI with contrast should be obtained. Additional imaging studies such as cerebral blood volume measures and MR spectroscopy can be considered if there is a diagnostic dilemma (single lesion, atypical location, atypical imaging features). LP studies should be obtained whenever leptomeningeal disease is suspected as positive cytology from the spinal fluid is the gold standard of diagnosing leptomeningeal disease. LP can also be pursued to assist in securing the diagnosis of parenchymal lesions, however, it has been estimated that only 10 percent of patients with metastases limited to the parenchyma have positive cytology (38). Hence, if there is a question of diagnosis, tissue sample via brain biopsy is likely required.

# Treatment

## Symptomatic Therapy

Therapy for brain metastases is divided into the immediate symptomatic therapies and "definitive therapies." If a patient is symptomatic and is found to have a brain mass associated with significant edema, glucocorticoids should be started immediately. Glucocorticoids are a mainstay of therapy for patients with metastatic brain tumors because they reduce the surrounding edema created by increased vasculature permeability in and around the tumor. Dexamethasone is often the steroid of choice, with doses ranging from 8–30mg/day in the acute period to 2–6mg/day maintenance, and tapered off as soon as clinically tolerated. Dexamethasone is often given intravenously at 10mg every 4–6 hours initially and then tapered after patients have achieved clinical improvement (often within 7–24 hours of the first dose). The lowest possible dose that provides symptom relief should be used as quickly as possible to reduce the chance of side effects from the glucocorticoids. That said, in general, steroid doses should not be changed any more frequently than every 5–7 days, as it takes that long to unmask neurologic deficits in the setting of a steroid taper.

Although steroids are rapidly active (within hours to days) and are often necessary for patients with tumor-related edema, they have many adverse effects that must be managed. These include irritable mood, mania and possible psychosis, sleep disruption, hyperglycemia, dyslipidemia, hypertension, and extremity swelling. Longer-term side effects are myopathy, gastritis, osteopenia, cushingoid features, and a relatively immunocompromised state that is particularly related to decreased CD4 counts. Hence, some advise prophylaxis for Pneumocystis pneumonia if patients will be on steroids for long periods of time (35). Patients are also advised to take proton pump inhibitors, calcium, and vitamin D supplements while on steroids to ameliorate the above-listed side effects.

Antiepileptic therapy is required only for patients who present with seizure. As discussed above, newer generation agents that do not interfere with hepatic metabolism are preferred. Appropriate analgesia should be provided to patients that present with headache. However, control of the ICP will often alleviate the headache pain and analgesic therapy can be minimized. In patients who have acute elevation in ICP, surgical interventions to relieve the pressure may be necessary. Otherwise, definitive therapy should be defined based on patients' clinical factors and wishes.

## Definitive Therapy

To date, even aggressive therapies have not resulted in a cure for most tumors that metastasize to brain. However, aggressive management may improve neurologic status and prolong survival in select cases. A patient's overall prognosis from the systemic cancer, the number of metastatic brain lesions, and the location of the lesions as well as patient performance status and prior therapies all have to be carefully considered. Therapeutic options include surgical resection, whole-brain radiation, focal radiation, radiosurgery and, increasingly, chemotherapy or a combination of the all of the above (52).

Surgery is usually the optimal approach for an accessible single lesion as it may significantly improve function and survival (46,53). Resection of the lesion may relieve tumor-associated mass effect, allowing for reduction or discontinuation of glucocorticoids (1). Surgery is also the optimal approach when the nature of the lesion is not entirely clear to secure diagnosis. Finally, surgery may be considered in the setting of multiple metastases if there is a lesion that is clearly causing symptoms that may be relieved with resection.

Whole brain radiation therapy (WBRT) is considered for patients who have multiple metastatic lesions or as a "consolidating" therapy after surgical resection. WBRT has been shown to increase the time to recurrence after surgical resection and reduce the incidence of death due to neurologic disease, but there is no difference in overall survival between patients who receive post-operative WBRT and those who do not (54). The choice to use WBRT must be weighed against the risk of neurologic sequelea. A study conducted at Memorial Sloan Kettering Cancer Center demonstrated that patients surviving one year or more after WBRT given at 10 fractions of 30 Gy had an 11 percent risk of dementia (55). Current dosing strategies give smaller fractions over longer time periods and correspondingly, the incidence of dementia appears to be lower. However, long-term cognitive deficits must be considered when discussing the benefits and risks of WBRT. There are also short-term side effects associated with WBRT including severe fatigue, memory loss, depression, transient worsening of neurologic symptoms, and hair loss that can negatively impact patient quality of life. That said, progression or recurrence of a tumor will also almost certainly negatively impact quality of life via worsening neurologic symptoms. Hence, a frank discussion of all of the potential risks and benefits of WBRT is advised to determine patient preference.

Stereotactic radiosurgery (SRS) is an increasingly popular therapy that can be used for both single and multiple metastases as long as the lesions are <4 cm (56,57). Although there are good responses with this therapy, it is not clear that SRS, with or without WBRT, improves survival. In general, some combination of surgery, SRS, and WBRT is commonly applied, especially to radiosensitive cancers such as small cell lung cancer and breast cancer.

Chemotherapy has traditionally been ineffective due to an inability of most agents to cross the blood brain barrier (BBB) and reach tumors. However, medications such as temozolomide and lapatinib have increasingly been tried in various forms of brain metastases with encouraging response rates and are currently undergoing formal investigation in clinical trials both as single agents and in combination therapy.

Temozolomide is an oral alkylating agent that is also a radiosentizer and is active against primary brain tumors such as glioblastoma multiforme. In brain metastases of various histologies, temozolomide monotherapy has had response rates of 4 to 10 percent (58,59). When added to WBRT, response rates increase to 31 to 96 percent (60–62).

Lapatinib is an oral small molecular tyrosine kinase inhibitor that targets ErbB2, ErbB1, HER2, and EGFR and has been demonstrated to have some efficacy against breast cancer brain metastases with 7.7 percent partial response and median time to progression of 16 weeks in heavily pretreated patients (63).

## Summary

Brain metastases are common among patients with systemic cancer and are a major source of morbidity and mortality. Timely recognition of neurologic symptoms that may be referable to a new brain metastasis may allow rapid stabilization of symptoms with interventions such as glucocorticoids. Options for definitive management are increasing and are generally well tolerated. This increasing number of therapeutic options for patients with brain metastases is encouraging, however, the overall survival remains relatively poor with an average of only 20 to 50 percent of patients alive one year after diagnosis. Often, the cause of death is progression of systemic metastases (54,64). Hence, the current goal of multimodality management of brain metastases is to minimize the tumor-associated symptoms, prevent neurologic progression, and, when systemic disease is well controlled, enhance survival. As therapeutics continue to improve, the importance of early recognition of brain metastases will become even more pertinent.

## References

1. Klos KJ, O'Neill BP. Brain metastases. *Neurologist* 2004;10:31–46.
2. Norden AD, Wen P, Kesari S. Brain Metastases. *Curr Opin Neurol* 2005;18:654–661.
3. Nguyen T, Abrey LE. Brain Metastases: Old problem, new strategies. *Hematol Oncol Clin North Am* 2007;21:369–388.
4. Richards GM, Khuntia D, Mehta MP. Therapeutic management of metastatic brain tumors. *Crit Rev Oncol Hematol* 2007;61:70-78.
5. Jaekle KA, Cohen ME, Duffner PK. Clinical presentations and therapy of nervous system tumors. In: Neurology in Clinical Practice. The Neurological Disorders. Bradley WG, Daroff RB, Fenichel GM, Marsden CD (Eds). Philadelphia: Butterwort Heinemann, 2000.
6. Grossman SA, Krabak MJ. Leptomeningeal carcinomatosis. *Cancer Treat Rev* 1999;25: 103–119.
7. Rasmussen BK. Epidemiology of Migraine. *Biomed Pharcother* 1995;49:452.
8. Christiaans MH, Kelder JC, Arnoldus EP, Tijssen CC. Prediction of intracranial metastases in cancer patients with headache. *Cancer* 2002;94:2063–2068.
9. Argyriou AA, Chroni E, Polychronopoulos P, Argyriou K, Papapetropoulos S, Corcondilas M, Lepoura N, Heras P. Headache characteristics and brain metastases prediction in cancer patients. *Eur J Cancer Care* 2006;15:90–95.
10. Forsyth PA, Posner JB. Headaches in patients with brain tumors: A study of 111 patients. *Neurology* 1993;43:1678–1683.
11. Kase CS. Intracerebral hemorrhage. In: Neurology in Clinical Practice. The Neurological Disorders. Bradley WG, Daroff RB, Fenichel GM, Marsden CD (Eds). Philadelphia: Butterwort Heinemann, 2000.
12. Glantz MJ, Cole BF, Forsyth PA, Recht LD, Wen PY, Chamberlain MC, Grossman SA, Cairncross JG. Practice Parameter: Anticonvulsant prophylaxis in patients with newly diagnosed brain tumors. Report of the Quality Standards Subcommittee on the American Academy of Neurology. *Neurology* 2000;54(10):1886–1893.
13. Lynam LM, Lyons MK, Drazkowski JF, Sirven JI, Noe KH, Zimmerman RS, Wilkens JA. Frequency of seizures in patients with newly diagnosed brain tumors: a retrospective review. *Clin Neurol Neurosurg* 2007;7:634–638.
14. Taillibert S, Delattre JY. Palliative care in patients with brain metastases. *Curr Opin Oncol* 2005;17:588–592.
15. Portenoy RK, Itri LM. Cancer-related fatigue: Guidelines for evaluation and management. *Oncologist* 1999;4:1–10.
16. Stone P, Richards M, A'Hern R, Hardy J. A study to investigate the prevalence, severity and correlates of fatigue among patients with cancer in comparison with a control group of volunteers without cancer. *Ann Oncol* 2000;11: 561–567.
17. Clouston PD, DeAngelis LM, Posner JB. The spectrum of neurologic disease in patients with systemic cancer. *Ann Neuro* 1992;31:268–273.
18. Tuma R, DeAngelis L. Altered mental status in patients with cancer. *Arch Neurol* 2000;57:1727–1731.
19. Siddiqi N, House AO, Holmes JD. Occurrence and outcome of delirium in medical in-patients: a systematic literature review. *Age Ageing* 2006;35:350–364.
20. Burstein HJ. Cognitive side-effects of adjuvant treatments. *Breast* 2007;16:166–168.
21. Ahles TA, Saykin AJ, Furstenberg CT, Cole B, Mott LA, Skalla K, Whedon MB, Bivens S, Mitchell T, Greenberg ER, Silberfarb PM. Neuropsychologic impact of standard-dose systemic chemotherapy in long-term survivors of breast cancer and lymphoma. *J Clin Oncol* 2002;20:485–493.

22. Schagen SB, van Dam FS, Muller MJ, Boogerd W, Lindeboom J, Bruning PF. Cognitive deficits after postoperative adjuvant chemotherapy for breast carcinoma. *Cancer* 1999;85:640–650.

23. O'Neill BP, Dinapoli RP, Okazaki H. Cerebral infarction as a result of tumor emboli. *Cancer* 1987;60:90–95.

24. Nolte, J. The Human Brain. An Introduction to Its Functional Anatomy. St Louis: Mosby, 1999.

25. Adolphs R, Tranel D, Hamann S, Young AW, Calder AJ, Phelps EA, Anderson A, Lee GP, Damasio AR. Recognition of facial emotion in nine individuals with bilateral amygdala damage. *Neuropsychologia* 1999;37:1111–1117.

26. Trimble MR, Mendez MF, Cummings JL. Neuropsychiatric symptoms from the temporolimbic lobes. *J Neuropsychiatry Clin Neurosci* 1997;9:429–438.

27. Ashwin PT, Tsaloumas MD. Complex visual hallucinations (Charles Bonnet syndrome) in the hemianopic visual field following occipital infarction. *J Neurol Sci* 2007;263:184–186.

28. Schmahmann J. Vascular syndromes of the thalamus. *Stroke* 2003;34: 2264–2278.

29. Carrera E, Bogousslavsky J. The thalamus and behavior: Effects of anatomically distinct strokes. *Neurology* 2006;66:1817–1823.

30. Misulis KE. Hemiplegia and monoplegia. In: Neurology in Clinical Practice. Principles of Diagnosis and Management. Bradley WG, Daroff RB, Fenichel GM, Marsden CD (Eds). Philadelphia: Butterwort Heinemann, 2000.

31. Darzy KH, Shalet SM. Hypopituitarism as a consequence of brain tumors and radiotherapy. *Pituitary* 2005;8:203–211.

32. Aaberg TM, Kay M, Sternau L. Metastatic tumors to the pituitary. *Am J Ophthalmol* 1995;119(6):779–785.

33. Juneau P, Schoene WC, Black P. Malignant tumors in the pituitary gland. *Arch Neurol* 1992;49:555–558.

34. Scheinberg D, Malslak P, Weiss M. Acute Leukemias In: DeVita V, Hellman S, Rosenberg S (Eds.) *Cancer: principles and practice of oncology*, 6th ed. Philadelphia: Lippincott Williams and Wilkins, 2001. pp. 2404–2433.

35. Taillibert S, Laigle-Donadey F, Chodkiewicz C, Sanson M, Hoang-Xuan K, Delattre JY. Leptomeningeal metastases from solid malignancy: a review. *J Neurooncol* 2005;75:85–99.

36. Wasserstrom WR, Glass JP, Posner JB. Diagnosis and treatment of leptomeningeal metastases from solid tumors: Experience with 90 patients. *Cancer* 1982;49:759–772.

37. Olson ME, Chernik NL, Posner JB. Infiltration of the leptomeninges by systemic cancer: A clinical and pathologic study. *Arch Neurol* 1974;30:122–137.

38. Balhuizen JC, Bots G, Schaberg A, Bosman F. Value of cerebrospinal fluid cytology for the diagnosis of malignancies in the central nervous system. *J Neurosurg* 1978;48:747–753.

39. Kaplan J, DeSouza T, Farkash A, Shafran B, Pack D, Rehman F, Fuks J, Portenoy R. Leptomeningeal metastases comparison of clinical features and laboratory data of solid tumors, lymphomas and leukemias. *J Neuro-Oncol* 1990;92:225–229.

40. Freilich RJ, Krol G, DeAngelis LM. Neuroimaging and cerebrospinal fluid cytology in the diagnosis of leptomeningeal metastasis. *Ann Neurol* 1995;38:51–57.

41. Straathof CS, de Bruin HG, Dippel DW, Vecht CJ. The diagnostic accuracy of magnetic resonance imaging and cerebrospinal fluid cytology in leptomeningeal metastasis. *J Neurol* 1999;246: 810–814.

42. Sze G, Milano E, Johnson C, Heier L. Detection of brain metastases: comparison of contrast-enhanced MR with unenhanced MR and enhanced CT. *AJNR Am J Neuroradiol* 1990;11:785–791.

43. Akeson P, Larsson EM, Kristoffersen DT, Jonsson E, Holtas S. Brain metastases—comparison of gadodiamide injection-enhanced MR imaging at standard and high dose, contrast-enhanced CT and non-contrast-enhanced MR imaging. *Acta Radiol* 1995;36:300–305.

44. Osburn AG. *Brain Tumors and Tumorlike Processes. Diagnostic Neuroradiology*. Patterson AS (Ed.). St. Louis: Mosby, 1994.

45. Gaviani P, M. M., Braga TA, Hedley-Whyte ET, Halpern EF, Schaefer PS, Henson JW. Improved detection of metastatic melanoma by T2*-weighted imaging. *AJNR Am J Neuroradiol* 2006;27(3):605–608.

46. Patchell RA, Tibbs PA, Walsh JW, Dempsey RJ, Maruyama Y, Kryscio RJ, Markesbery WR, Macdonald JS, Young B. A randomized trial of surgery in the treatment of single metastases to the brain. *N Engl J Med* 1990;322:494–500.

47. Forsyth PA, Kelly PJ, Cascino TL, Scheithauer BW, Shaw EG, Dinapoli RP, Atkinson EJ. Radiation necrosis or glioma recurrence: is computer-assisted stereotactic biopsy useful? *J Neurosurg* 1995;82:436–444.

48. Nelson SJ. Multivoxel magnetic resonance spectroscopy of brain tumors. *Mol Cancer Ther* 2003;2:497–507.

49. Rees J. Advances in magnetic resonance imaging of brain tumours. *Curr Opin Neurol* 2003;16:643–650.

50. Chiang IC, Kuo YT, Lu CY, Yeung KW, Lin WC, Sheu FO, Liu GC. Distinction between high-grade gliomas and solitary metastases using peritumoral 3-T magnetic resonance spectroscopy, diffusion, and perfusion imagings. *Neuroradiology* 2004;46:619–627.

51. Chen W. Clinical applications of PET in brain tumors. *J Nucl Med* 2007;48:1468–1481.

52. Soffietti R, Rudç R, Mutani R. Management of brain metastases. *J Neurol* 2002;249:1357–1369.

53. Vecht CJ, Haaxma-Reiche H, Noordijk EM, Padberg GW, Voormolen JH, Hoekstra FH, Tans JT, Lambooij N, Metsaars JA, Wattendorff AR, et al. Treatment of single brain metastasis: Radiotherapy alone or combined with neurosurgery? *Ann Neurol* 1993;33:583–590.

54. Patchell RA, Tibbs PA, Regine WF, Dempsey RJ, Mohiuddin M, Kryscio RJ, Markesbery WR, Foon KA, Young B. Postoperative radiotherapy in the treatment of single metastases to the brain: a randomized trial. *JAMA* 1998;280:1485–1489.

55. DeAngelis L, Delattre JY, Posner JB. Radiation-induced dementia in patients cured of brain metastases. *Neurology* 1989;39:789–796.

56. Martin JJ, Kondziolka D.Indications for resection and radiosurgery for brain metastases. *Curr Opin Oncol* 2005;17:584–587.

57. Mehta MP, Tsao MN, Whelan TJ, Morris DE, Hayman JA, Flickinger JC, Mills M, Rogers CL, Souhami L. The American Society for Therapeutic Radiology and Oncology (ASTRO) evidence-based review of the role of radiosurgery for brain metastases. *Int J Radiation Oncology Biol* Phys 2005;63:37–46.

58. Abrey LE, Olson JD, Raizer JJ, Mack M, Rodavitch A, Boutros DY, Malkin MG. A phase II trial of temozolomide for patients with recurrent or progressive brain metastases. *J Neurooncol* 2001;53(3):259–265.

59. Agarwala SS, Kirkwood JM, Gore M, Dreno B, Thatcher N, Czarnetski B, Atkins M, Buzaid A, Skarlos D, Rankin EM. Temozolomide for the treatment of brain metastases associated with metastatic melanoma: a phase II study. *J Clin Oncol* 2004;22:2101–2107.

60. Giorgio CG, Giuffrida D, Pappalardo A, Russo A, Santini D, Salice P, Blanco G, Castorina S, Failla G, Bordonaro R. Oral temozolomide in heavily pre-treated brain metastases from non-small cell lung cancer: phase II study. *Lung Cancer* 2005;50:247–254.

61. Biswas G, Bhagwat R, Khurana R, Menon H, Prasad N, Parikh PM. Brain metastasis—evidence based management. *J Cancer Res Ther* 2006;2:5–13.

62. Addeo R, Caraglia M, Faiola V, Capasso E, Vincenzi B, Montella L, Guarrasi R, Caserta L, Del Prete S. Concomitant treatment of brain metastasis with whole brain radiotherapy [WBRT] and temozolomide [TMZ] is active and improves quality of life. BMC *Cancer* 2007;25;7:18.

63. Lin NU, Dieras V, Paul D, Lossignol D, Christodoulou C, Laessig D, Roché H, Zembryki D, Oliva CR, Winer EP. (2007) EGF105084 Study Group. EGF105084, a phase II study of lapatinib for brain metastases in patients (pts) with HER2+ breast cancer following trastuzumab (H) based systemic therapy and cranial radiotherapy (RT). *J Clin Oncol*, 2007 ASCO Annual Meeting Proceedings Part I. Vol. 25, No. 18S (June 20 Supplement):1012.

64. Wadasadawala T, Gupta S, Bagul V, Patil N. Brain metastases from breast cancer: management approach. *J Cancer Res Ther* 2007;3:157–165.

# 2

# Radiation Therapy for Brain Metastases

James B. Yu

Jonathan P.S. Knisely

Brain metastases are common in patients with advanced cancer. In adults, brain metastases occur up to 10 times as frequently as primary brain tumors, are the most common intracranial malignancy, and are found in 15 to 30 percent of autopsies of all cancer patients (1–3). In children, however, brain metastases occur less frequently than primary brain tumors (4,5). Estimates for the incidence of brain metastases in the United States range from 60,000 to 170,000 cases per year (6,7). Usual therapeutic options for patients with brain metastases include surgical resection, stereotactic radiosurgery, and whole-brain radiation. Whole-brain radiation is a frequently administered treatment, and in patients with disseminated or unresectable disease, whole brain radiation therapy remains a primary treatment for intracranial metastatic disease (8). Whole-brain radiation is also given before or after more focal and directed treatments, such as surgery or stereotactic radiosurgery.

In terms of overall incidence, the most frequent primary tumors causing brain metastases are lung cancer, breast cancer, melanoma, colorectal cancer, renal cell carcinoma, testicular cancer, thyroid cancer, and cancer of unknown primary origin (6,9,10). Survival after treatment for brain metastases varies, but brain metastases are almost invariably an indicator of incurable disease. Untreated symptomatic patients have a median survival of less than 7 weeks (10).

## Pathogenesis

Metastases are thought to occur when the primary tumor acquires the ability to migrate and grow elsewhere. This involves the completion of a sequence of steps, involving the intravasation of cells from the primary tumor, travel of the cells in the circulation (either lymphatic or hematologic or both), movement from the circulation into the distant organ (extravasation), and the initiation and maintenance of tumor proliferation in the metastatic site (11).

The brain is a unique environment for metastases. Because of the continuously connected endothelium surrounding the brain, which is known as the blood-brain barrier, it is thought to be a sanctuary site from chemotherapy. The endothelium is connected with tight junctions, surrounded by astrocytes and pericytes and a basement membrane, and loaded with efflux pumps (11). The blood-brain barrier severely curtails the movement of macromolecules from the blood stream into the brain (12). The tendency of certain primary tumors to metastasize to the brain involves both primary tumor and target (brain) characteristics (11). Hematogenous metastases to the brain parenchyma tend to occur at the gray-white junction (64 percent) and at the border zone regions of the cerebral vascular supply (62 percent). This is theorized to result from the sudden narrowing of arteriolar diameters as they enter the white matter, causing tumor microemboli to lodge at the gray-white matter junction. The terminal capillary beds of cerebral arteries are also suspected potential sites for tumor emboli impaction and seeding (13).

## Diagnosis

Symptoms from brain metastases are dependent on the location, size, and number of metastases. Patients can be completely asymptomatic and have metastases appear on imaging alone, or they may have seizures and experience severe incapacitation. Brain metastases can be diagnosed at staging work-up for the primary tumor or be discovered after active cancer therapy.

Symptoms of brain metastases include headache, weakness, mental status changes, slurred speech, seizure, coordination difficulties, visual field deficits, and other sensory disturbances. Headache is the most common symptom (14).

Studies report that 75 to 85 percent of lesions are supratentorial only, and when detected by computed-tomography (CT) scan, approximately 50 percent of brain metastases are single lesions (3,10,14). Magnetic resonance imaging (MRI) is more sensitive in the detection of brain metastases than CT, and the proportion of patients with single lesions is likely closer to one-fifth than to one-third (15–18). Thirty-one percent of patients with brain metastases found on CT scan who were thought to have only single metastases actually had multiple brain metastases (15). Impressively, MRI imaging findings have led to earlier detection of brain metastases, often before symptoms have become manifest. Because of this, contrast enhanced MRI is the gold standard for detection of brain metastases (13). Double or triple dose MRI will reveal additional brain metastases, and high resolution volumetric acquisitions will also increase the detection of brain metastases (13,19–21).

## Description of Treatment Modalities

Although corticosteroids can extend survival by several weeks (22), modern treatment of brain metastases relies on various combinations of surgery, stereotactic radiosurgery, and whole-brain radiation. Concerns about chemotherapy access to the central nervous system (CNS) have precluded use of this approach for managing most brain metastases. The use of chemotherapy for systemic disease is likely to have some beneficial effects in certain clinical scenarios, but it must still be regarded as largely investigational for brain metastases relative to well-established roles for surgery, radiosurgery, and radiation therapy. The following sections describe radiotherapeutic technique in general terms and then outline the rationale behind various treatment recommendations for patients with cancer metastatic to the brain. To aid in clinical decision making, the major randomized trials (Table 2.1) and treatment recommendations (Table 2.2) are shown.

### Whole-Brain Radiation

Whole-brain radiation is usually delivered with the patient lying supine, with the head immobilized to minimize movement during treatment and to maximize position reproducibility (Figure 2.1). The head is usually immobilized using a perforated thermoplastic mask that is shaped to conform to the individual patient's facial features. Treatment is usually less than 15 minutes in duration, and this time frame includes bringing the patient into the treatment room, positioning the patient, verifying field position with electronic portal imaging, administering treatment, and helping the patient off the treatment table. Typical "beam-on" time is less than 3 or 4 minutes.

Whole-brain radiation treatment portals encompass the entire brain, and treatment is typically administered with two opposed helmet-shaped radiation fields, delivered with several degree couch rotations to make the beam edges

TABLE 2.1 Randomized Trials of Various Management Strategies in Patients with Brain Metastases—Reported Overall Survival

| | WBRT | WBRT + SRS | SRS | SURGERY | SURGERY + WBRT | P VALUE |
|---|---|---|---|---|---|---|
| Andrews et al. (66) (n=333) | 6.5 months | 5.7 months | | | | 0.1356 |
| Kondziolka et al. (67) (n=27) | 7.5 months | 11 months | | | | 0.22 |
| Chougule et al. (68) (n=96) | 9 months | 5 months | 7 months | | | Nonsig. |
| Patchell et al. (42) (n=95) | | | | 9.9 months* | 11.1 months* | 0.39 |
| Aoyama et al. (62) (n=132) | | 7.5 months | 8 months | | | 0.42 |
| Vecht et al. (43)/ Noordijk et al.(45) (n=63) | 6 months | | | | 10 months | 0.04 |
| Patchell et al. (48) (n=48) | 3.5 months* | | | | 9.2 months* | <0.01 |
| Mintz et al. (44) (n=84) | 6.3 months | | | | 5.6 months | 0.24 |

*Converted from weeks (reported number) to months, with 4 1/3 weeks = 1 month.

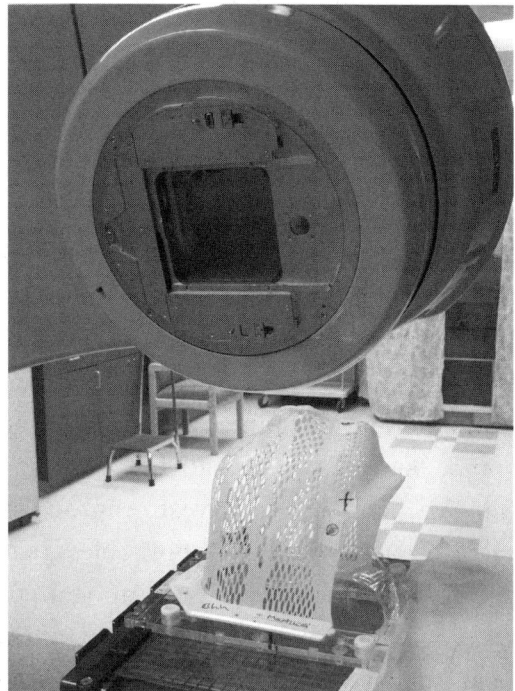

FIGURE 2.1   A thermoplastic mask and linear accelerator. For WBRT treatment, a patient typically lies supine, with head immobilized by a mask. The linear accelerator treats from one side of the brain and then the other.

TABLE 2.2  Treatment Recommendation

| RTOG RPA CLASS | NUMBER OF METASTASES | RECOMMENDATION | RATIONALE | STRENGTH OF RECOMMENDATION** |
|---|---|---|---|---|
| I | 1 | Surgical resection and WBRT if possible rather than WBRT. | Patchell et al. (42) and Noordijk et al. (45)/ Vecht et al. (43) showed a survival benefit to surgery and WBRT versus WBRT alone. Mintz et al. did not show a survival benefit. | Class I (Evidence from at least one properly designed randomized controlled trial) |
| | | | In addition, surgery provides for immediate debulking and symptom relief in comparison to WBRT alone. Quality of life is maintained much longer than in patients treated with radiation alone. | |
| | | Alternately, SRS and WBRT are preferred over WBRT alone. | Andrews et al. (66) showed improvement in local control with the addition of SRS to WBRT. | Class I |
| | | | Andrews et al. (66) in subset analysis, showed that for patients with a single brain metastasis, there is an improvement in survival for SRS + WBRT versus WBRT alone. Other retrospective studies, Sanghavi et al. (64), also demonstrated this. | Based on unplanned subset analysis of Class I evidence, and Class II-3 |
| | | After surgical resection, WBRT recommended rather than surgical resection alone. | Patchell et al. (48) showed no survival benefit with addition of WBRT up-front, but improvement in prevention of neurologic death, and intracranial control benefit. | Class I |
| | | After SRS, WBRT is to be strongly considered to decrease intracranial recurrence. | Chougule et al.(68), Aoyama et al. (62), noted no survival difference in SRS versus SRS + WBRT, but intracranial relapse occurred more frequently with the omission of WBRT. | Class I |

(continued on next page)

TABLE 2.2 Treatment Recommendation (continued)

| RTOG RPA CLASS | NUMBER OF METASTASES | RECOMMENDATION | RATIONALE | STRENGTH OF RECOMMENDATION** |
|---|---|---|---|---|
| | | SRS versus Surgery + WBRT | Muacevic et al. (54) found equivalent local control after SRS and with WBRT + SRS in comparison to surgery. | Class II-2 |
| I | 2-3 (or 2-4) | SRS + WBRT preferred over WBRT alone. | For 1-3 metastases, Andrews et al. (66) showed improved local control. In addition, for 1-3 metastases and RPA Class I, Andrews et al. on unplanned subset analysis showed there was also a survival benefit. Kondziolka et al. (67) showed improved control of brain disease for 2-4 metastases. | Class I |
| | | After SRS, WBRT is to be strongly considered to prevent intracranial recurrence. | Chougule et al. (68) and Aoyama et al. (62) noted no survival difference in SRS versus SRS + WBRT, but intracranial relapse occurred more frequently with the omission of WBRT. Survival is not affected by the early delivery of WBRT. | Class I |
| I | 4+ | SRS + WBRT may be considered in patients with a low aggregate volume of metastatic disease. | Retrospective series by Bhatnagar et al. (71) show improvement in survival compared to historical control. | Class II-3 |
| | 4+ | WBRT may be considered in all patients | WBRT increases overall survival in comparison to corticosteroids alone, and decreases the rate of intracranial disease progression. | Class II-2, II-3 |
| | | | In patients with excellent functional status with longer expected survival, it is reasonable to use a more prolonged fractionation scheme (such as 2 Gy x 20 fractions). Although no survival benefit has been demonstrated, theoretically, smaller fraction sizes will reduce long term toxicity. | Class III |

TABLE 2.2 Treatment Recommendation (continued)

| RTOG RPA CLASS | NUMBER OF METASTASES | RECOMMENDATION | RATIONALE | STRENGTH OF RECOMMENDATION** |
|---|---|---|---|---|
| I–III | 1, 2, 3 or 4+ | SRS alone as initial treatment | Sneed et al. (59) identified improved intracranial control, but no improved survival for RPA Classes I–III, in patients with the addition of WBRT to SRS (SRS versus SRS WBRT for RPA Class I–III was 14.0 versus 15.2 m; 8.2 versus 7.0 m; 5.3 versus 5.5 m., p=0.33). Shu et al. (128) also observed no benefit in overall survival for patients who receive SRS alone versus historical experience in patients treated with WBRT + SRS. | Class II-2 |
| II | 1 | SRS and WBRT preferred over WBRT alone. | Andrews et al. (66) included patients with RPA Class II. As noted above, on unplanned subset analysis there was a slight survival benefit to SRS + WBRT over WBRT alone. | Unplanned subset analysis of Class I data. |
| | 1 | Surgery + WBRT preferred over WBRT alone, and over surgery alone. | In both studies by Patchell et al. (42,48) patients in RPA class II were included. | Class I |
| | 2–3 (or 1–4) | SRS and WBRT preferred over WBRT alone. | Patients with oligometastases may still benefit from SRS, even if in RPA Class II. Kondziolka et al. (67) included RPA Class II patients, and although a survival benefit was not found overall, in patients who strictly had WBRT alone (excluding patients who had delayed SRS salvage for recurrence) compared to up front SRS + WBRT, there was a survival benefit to SRS + WBRT. Andrews et al. (66) also included RPA Class II patients. | Class II-3 |
| | | After SRS, WBRT to be strongly considered to decrease risk of intracranial relapse. | Aoyama et al. (62) included RPA Class II patients. | Class I |

*(continued on next page)*

TABLE 2.2 Treatment Recommendation (continued)

| RTOG RPA CLASS | NUMBER OF METASTASES | RECOMMENDATION | RATIONALE | STRENGTH OF RECOMMENDATION** |
|---|---|---|---|---|
| | 4+ | SRS and WBRT may be considered versus WBRT alone. | Nam et al. (70) and Bhatnagar et al. (71), in retrospective series, showed prolonged survival for RPA Class II patients with 4+ lesions who received SRS + WBRT in comparison to historical controls of patients who received WBRT. Neider et al. (129), however, did not demonstrate a correlation between RPA classification and survival. | Class II-3, III |
| III | Any | WBRT. | WBRT has been shown to improve survival over corticosteroids alone, and decrease the rate of intracranial progression. | Class III |
| | | Corticosteroids or supportive care alone may be considered in patients expected to survive <8 weeks after the end of proposed WBRT treatment. | The identification of patients who would not benefit from WBRT (patients for whom steroids alone provide good neurologic palliation, and systemic disease will likely cause death before 8 weeks) is still problematic (130). WBRT should only be omitted after an informed discussion with the patient and family regarding short term and long-term goals of care, and pros and cons of WBRT treatment or omission. WBRT remains the standard of care for all patients with symptomatic brain metastases. | |

SRS ± WBRT rationales based on recommendations from Mehta MP, Tsao MN, Whelan TJ, et al. The American Society for Therapeutic Radiology and Oncology (ASTRO) evidence-based review of the role of radiosurgery for brain metastases. *Int J Radiat Oncol Biol Phys* 2005;63:37-46. Other recommendations are generated by the authors.

\*   Use caution with tumor size greater than 3 cm.

\*\*  Class I – Evidence obtained from at least one properly designed randomized controlled trial.

    Class II-1 – Evidence obtained from well-designed controlled trial, not randomized

    Class II-2 – Evidence obtained form well-designed cohort or case-control analytic studies, preferably from more than one center or group

    Class II-3 – Evidence obtained from comparisons between times or places with or without the intervention

    Class III – Opinions of respected authorities, based on clinical experience, descriptive studies or reports of expert committees.

coplanar behind the lenses of the eyes and collimator rotations to facilitate a clear junction plane between the bottom of the radiotherapy portal and the adjacent cervical vertebral body. Traditionally, whole-brain radiation has been given using rectangular fields angled so that the inferior border of the field encompasses the bony orbit and foramen magnum (Figure 2.2). Helmet-field irradiation utilizes lead blocks or multileaf collimators (Figure 2.3), which shape the field to prevent irradiating anterior structures unnecessarily and provide better coverage of the entire brain and meninges (Figure 2.4).

Commonly utilized fractionation schemes for whole-brain radiation for existing metastases or prophylaxis include 40 Gy in 20 fractions, 37.5 Gy in 15 fractions, 36 Gy in 18 fractions, 30 Gy in 10 or 15 fractions, and 20 Gy in 5 fractions. Lower fraction sizes are not associated with an increased risk of late toxicity (23). Higher radiation fraction sizes, as noted in the previous chapter, have been associated with higher rates of dementia. DeAngelis et al., in a highly cited paper (24), reported a high rate of dementia (11 percent) in long-term survivors of whole brain radiation therapy (WBRT), likely caused by the larger fraction sizes used during that time (4 to 8 Gy) compared to the currently accepted standard (2 to 3 Gy). The possible contribution of chemotherapy or other factors, including systemic disease progression, was not assessed.

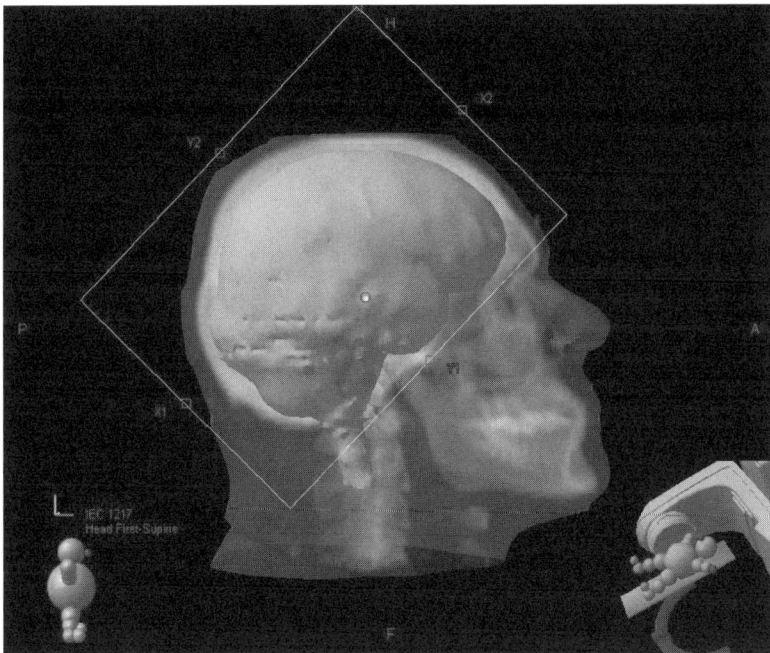

FIGURE 2.2   Typical whole-brain radiotherapy field.

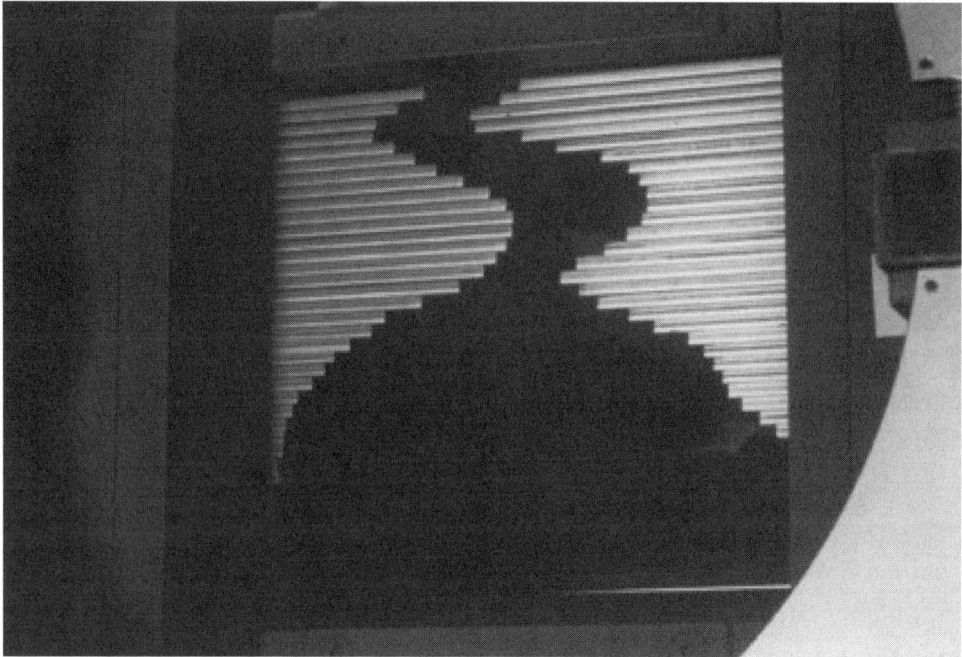

FIGURE 2.3   Typical multileaf collimator, used to shape the beam. Photo courtesy of Elekta.

In the patients irradiated at lower fraction sizes, the toxicity level was more acceptable. The effect of fraction size has been demonstrated in patients who have undergone radiotherapy for low-grade gliomas, suggesting that cognitive

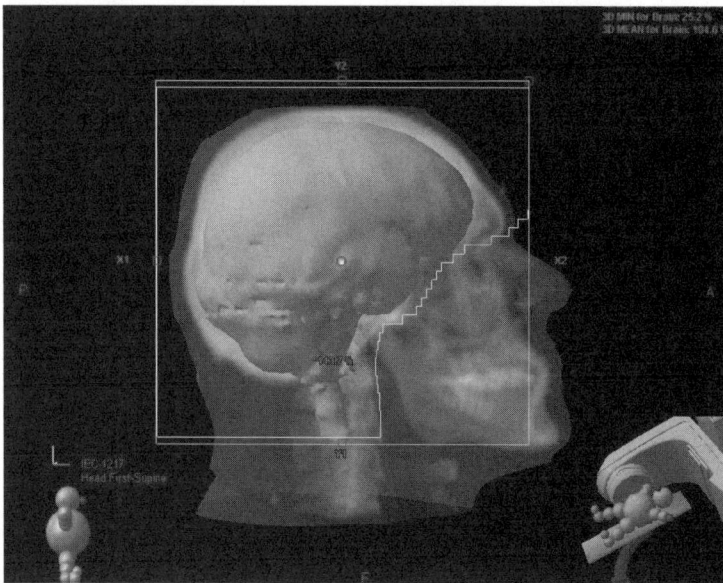

FIGURE 2.4   A typical helmet field, encompassing all brain and spinal cord to the bottom of the C2 vertebral body.

disability and deleterious sequelae from radiotherapy occur more frequently when high fraction doses (greater than 2 Gy) are used (25). The most commonly delivered fractionation scheme is 30 Gy in 10 fractions, and this dose fractionation scheme is widely considered the current standard for WBRT (26).

Numerous schedules for WBRT, ranging from 10 to 54 Gy in 1 to 34 fractions, have been studied by the Radiation Therapy Oncology Group (RTOG) (Table 2.3) in randomized trials (27,28). All fractionation schemes studied were equivalent with respect to overall toxicity, neurologic improvement, and survival, but higher fraction sizes were associated with greater neurologic toxicity (29,30). For patients with greater prospects of long-term survival, it is reasonable to use a more prolonged fractionation scheme to try to minimize late toxicity because of the radiobiological effect of high fraction sizes on late responding tissues in the CNS (24,31).

Corticosteroid therapy is often administered concurrently with whole-brain radiotherapy to decrease cerebral edema, but it may not be needed if there is no significant mass effect or edema visualized on the diagnostic imaging studies.

Metastatic histologies typically excluded from trials involving whole-brain radiation alone include leukemia, lymphoma, and germ cell tumors, because of their usual rapid response to radiotherapy. Melanoma and renal cell carcinomas, because of their relative radioresistance, are increasingly treated with stereotactic radiosurgery alone as initial treatment (or with surgical resec-

TABLE 2.3 Randomized Trials by the RTOG Involving Different Fractionation Schemes for Whole-Brain Radiation

| AUTHOR | FRACTIONATION SCHEME | SURVIVAL | P VALUE |
|---|---|---|---|
| Borgelt et al. 1980 (39) | 40 Gy (20 fx) <br> 40 Gy (15 fx) <br> 30 Gy (15 fx) <br> 30 Gy (10 fx) <br> 20 Gy (5 fx) | 3.2–4.6 months | >0.05 |
| Borgelt et al. 1981 (132) | 30–40 Gy (10–20 fx) <br> 20 Gy (5 fx) <br> 12 Gy (2 fx) <br> 10 Gy (1 fx) | 2.8–4.8 months | >0.05 |
| Kurtz et al. 1981 (133) | 50 Gy (20 fx) <br> 30 Gy (10 fx) | 4.0–4.4 months | >0.05 |
| Murray et al. 1997 (134) | 54.4 Gy (34 fx–BID) <br> 30 Gy (10 fx) | 4.5 months | >0.05 |

tion in appropriate cases), with whole-brain radiation reserved for multiple metastases or symptomatic metastases requiring immediate treatment that are not amenable to surgery (32–35).

## Stereotactic Radiosurgery

Stereotactic radiosurgery is a focused form of radiation treatment. Typically, radiation is delivered via a treatment machine with multiple simultaneous convergent beams to a single focus point (Leksell Gamma Knife), or with a precisely targeted linear accelerator (Linac) that delivers multiple sequential convergent beams, or by using an arcing beam with a precise focal point (Linac based stereotactic radiosurgery). Charged-particle (proton and carbon ion) therapy can also be used in a manner similar to that used with a conventional linear accelerator, though there are significant differences in the physics and radiobiology of charged-particle treatment.

Stereotaxis is traditionally determined by a fixed alignment of the patient to a physical coordinate system, either a stereotactic headframe or other equivalent immobilization device. There are now devices that are capable of ensuring acceptable accuracy for many indications without affixing a headframe to the patient's skull. The discussion of the pros and cons of different immobilization devices and treatment machines is beyond the scope of this chapter, but it is important to note that there is no strong clinical data that suggests superiority of one or another platform for stereotactic radiosurgery (SRS) as regards lesion control and patient outcome, and all machines can be considered equally appropriate with proper administration and immobilization.

# Rationale for Choosing Treatment

## Whole-Brain Radiation Alone

Whole-brain radiation therapy is effective at reducing intracranial metastasis growth (8,10), and is associated with prolonging survival (36,37). Response rates to treatment are high, with an improvement in neurologic function in >60 percent of patients. Two-thirds of these patients will have long-lasting neurologic symptom relief (7). Unfortunately, cranial nerve deficits are often refractory, and only 40 percent of patients experience any measurable improvement (7). Median survival for patients treated with WBRT is 2.3 to 7.1 months, depending on performance status, age, and disease state (38). Whole-brain radiation is often given alone to patients who are not appropriate candidates for stereotactic radiosurgery or surgical resection, and is also often used in combination with these treatments.

Neurologic symptoms from regrowth of metastatic foci may recur in patients treated with WBRT if they survive long enough; the median time to progression for all patients with brain metastases is only 2–3 months after WBRT (39). Because of this, and because neurosurgical resection can alleviate symptoms from mass effect and makes it possible to obtain a tissue diagnosis (if this is uncertain), resection of an isolated metastatic focus has long been used for patients with brain metastasis as a way of improving intracranial control beyond what is possible with WBRT alone.

## Surgical Resection With or Without Whole-Brain Radiation

Surgical resection has been used for decades with patients requiring immediate decompression of a large metastasis as well as for radiographically identified and easily accessible, isolated lesions. Because of its efficacy at relieving mass effect and achieving local control, it is arguably the standard of care for these patients. Surgical resection, especially of the posterior fossa or large or radiore-sistant tumors, improves intracranial hypertension and allows for a more rapid tapering of corticosteroids (40,41).

Two randomized trials have confirmed the benefits of surgical resection in patients with a single metastasis and good performance status when compared to treatment by whole-brain radiation alone (42,43). Another randomized trial, however, did not confirm this hypothesis (44).

The first trial supporting surgical resection was reported by Patchell et al. (42). Forty-eight patients with a single metastasis and Karnofsky performance status (KPS) ≥70 (recursive partitioning analysis [RPA] Class I and II) were randomly chosen for resection with WBRT or stereotactic biopsy with WBRT. Patients were given dexamethasone 4 mg every 6 hours, which was continued through radiation. WBRT was 3 Gy $\times$ 12 fractions for a total of 36 Gy. Resection and postoperative WBRT resulted in better local control (20 percent local recurrence versus 52 percent local recurrence, p<0.02). Time to recurrence was also improved with resection (>59 weeks versus 21 weeks, p<0.0001). Median survival was improved (40 weeks versus 15 weeks, p<0.01), but risk from systemic death did not change. Quality of life was also much improved (patients maintained a KPS >70 for a median of 38 weeks for the resection group versus 8 weeks, p<0.005 for patients not treated with resection). There was significant reduction in mortality from neurologic causes (62 weeks versus 26 weeks, p<0.0009). Interestingly, 11 percent of the patients enrolled in this study (6 of 54) with radiographically diagnosed brain metastases seen on contrast CT or MRI were not histologically diagnosed with brain metastases. Three of these patients had potentially reversible infectious or inflammatory conditions.

This raises an important point that biopsy or resection to confirm the nature of a lesion is especially important in patients with controlled extracranial disease. For these patients, survival and quality of life may well depend on appropriate treatment of the brain lesion.

The second trial supporting microsurgical resection was published by Vecht et al. (43) and was later republished by Noordijk et al. (45). Sixty-three patients were randomly selected for surgery and WBRT versus WBRT alone. A greater survival benefit was observed for the surgery + WBRT group compared to the WBRT only group (10 months versus 6 months, p=0.04). The WBRT used 2 Gy bid × 2 weeks, for a total dose of 40 Gy. Minimum interfraction time was only 4 hours. This accelerated fractionation was well tolerated, and at the time of reporting, 9 long-term survivors had not manifested late neurological side effects (such as dementia) from the radiation, but a detailed psychologic assessment was not performed as part of the study. In addition, maintenance of functional independence improved, though this improvement was not statistically significant (7.5 months versus 3.5 months, p=0.06). For patients without active extracranial disease, median survival was 12 months versus 7 months favoring the surgery + WBRT arm versus WBRT alone. This was the subset group with the greatest benefit.

Mintz et al. (44) conducted a randomized study with 84 patients for surgery + WBRT versus WBRT alone. Unlike in the two prior randomized trials, there was no significant difference in median survival (6.3 months versus 5.6 months, p=0.24). This trial was complicated by the fact that resection was incomplete in 10 percent of patients, and approximately 25 percent of patients randomized to WBRT alone also had surgery. The contradictory nature of the Mintz trial may also be partially due to a lower KPS for the study population in comparison to study populations in the Patchell and Vecht trials, and a higher proportion of patients who also had extracranial metastases.

Based on the evidence from the randomized trials and retrospective data noted above, in patients with single metastases and KPS >70, controlled primary tumor, absence of extracranial metastases, and age <65 (RTOG RPA Class I), a strong recommendation can be made for using surgical resection in conjunction with WBRT rather than using WBRT alone. Indeed, for single-brain metastases, surgical resection still remains a standard of care.

The question then arises: Can surgery be used without WBRT? Two retrospective studies found no survival advantage to adjuvant WBRT (46,47). Although an increased rate of dementia was perceived with adjuvant WBRT, larger radiation fraction sizes than are commonly used in modern treatment were used in these studies.

Patchell and his colleagues at the University of Kentucky performed another landmark randomized trial that focused on this question (48). Ninety-five patients with single metastases to the brain after a complete surgical resection received adjuvant WBRT or no immediate therapy (with radiation allowed for salvage). The completeness of surgical resection was verified by MRI. Radiotherapy was started within 28 days of surgery, and radiosensitive primary tumors (small cell lung cancer, germ cell tumors, lymphoma, leukemia, and multiple myeloma) were excluded. Patients treated with WBRT received 50.4 Gy in 28 1.8 Gy fractions over 5.5 weeks. The primary endpoint of this study was to determine recurrence rates of tumor in the brain. Secondary endpoints included the assessment of survival, cause of death, and preservation of ability to function independently. WBRT predictably prevented intracranial recurrence (18 versus 70 percent, p<0.001) and other metastatic disease in the brain (14 versus 37 percent, p<0.01). Local control at the site of resection was also improved (recurrence rate 10 percent versus 46 percent, p<0.001). Overall survival was not affected (48 versus 43 weeks), but death from neurologic causes was less frequent in the cohort getting adjuvant WBRT (14 percent versus 44 percent). Unfortunately, patients in the WBRT group were more likely to die of systemic cancer rather than neurologic progression, and so the authors hypothesized that the absence of a difference in overall survival between the two treatment arms was a result of the lack of satisfactory treatment for the systemic cancers and not due to a failure of postoperative radiotherapy to control the disease in the brain. The duration of functional independence was not altered by the addition of WBRT to surgical resection.

Based on this clinical trial, postoperative WBRT can be recommended for patients who have undergone surgical resection of an isolated brain metastasis, with the expectation that local control will be improved and death from neurologic causes will be less frequent.

## Surgical Resection versus Stereotactic Radiosurgery

There have been no completed phase III trials comparing microsurgical resection and stereotactic radiosurgery. Both are focal therapies, and when used for metastatic cancer, neither can address metastases that are not specifically targeted. Surgery also affords the possibility of a tissue diagnosis. Retrospective comparative analyses of efficacy and economics have been performed for stereotactic radiosurgery and resection, and radiosurgery is more cost effective than surgical resection (41,49).

Stereotactic radiosurgery has emerged as an effective and precise method of delivering focused radiation, which avoids the expected sequelae from whole-brain radiotherapy (50–52). Stereotactic radiosurgery is relatively safe with careful patient selection, though with increasing numbers of tumors and tumor volume there is an associated increased risk of short- and long-term sequelae (52). RTOG 9005 was a phase I study that attempted to define the safest tolerable radiosurgery dose for recurrent primary brain tumors and metastases <2 cm, 2–3 cm and >3–4 cm in size following conventional irradiation. In a multivariate analysis of the entire cohort, compared to tumors <20 mm in maximum diameter, 21–30 mm tumors had a 7.3 times higher risk of developing unacceptable CNS toxicity, and 31–40 mm tumors had a 16 times higher risk (52). An infrequent complication from stereotactic radiosurgery is radionecrosis, sometimes requiring resection and sometimes resulting in death. A range of incidence of operation rates for radionecrosis has been reported from <1 percent of patients treated (50) with an increase up to 11 percent at 2 years (52). Radionecrosis rates are higher with larger doses given to larger lesions (51). However, lowering the radiosurgical dose for larger lesions decreases the local control rate (51). Other possible side effects include periprocedural seizures, delayed cerebral edema requiring steroids, and (rarely) a hemorrhagic stroke from bleeding into a metastasis.

Interestingly, in RTOG 9005, in addition to higher tumor sizes, a higher KPS predicted a higher risk of unacceptable CNS toxicity (52). Improved local control (95 percent) for higher doses (>20Gy) are also associated with a higher level of RTOG grade 4 toxicity: 5.9 percent for >20Gy (53).

Muacevic et al. performed a population matched retrospective study comparing surgery + WBRT to radiosurgery alone as primary treatment for solitary cerebral metastasis (54). Eligibility criteria included having a single metastasis <3.5 cm in size. Fifty-two patients were observed as having had surgery + WBRT, and 56 patients had SRS alone as up-front treatment. There was a statistically insignificant shorter overall survival observed in the SRS-alone group. One year survival for surgery + WBRT versus SRS was 53 percent versus 43 percent (p=0.19), and median survival for surgery + WBRT versus SRS was 68 weeks versus 35 weeks (p=0.19). Shorter overall survival in the SRS-alone group was attributed to higher systemic death rates. Remote intracranial control was worse with the omission of WBRT. Neurological death rates were the same. The conclusion of the authors was that SRS was the same as surgery + WBRT in selected patients, and that for selected patients treated with SRS, WBRT was not needed.

Several significant differences exist between a microsurgical resection of a brain metastasis and the radiosurgical treatment of a brain metastasis, and consideration of these differences may help guide treatment recommendations for individual patients. The benefit of obtaining histopathological confirmation of a pathological process is only possible with surgery, as stated above, and immediate relief of mass effect is only possible with a microsurgical approach.

A gross total microsurgical resection of a brain metastasis often leaves microscopic disease at the edge of the resection cavity. This likely explains the high rate of local recurrence after surgery alone (48). No antitumor effect occurs beyond the plane of resection. In contrast, a radiosurgical procedure will have a penumbra of dose extending beyond the prescription isodose surface, which will treat microscopic extension of disease beyond the visible margin of the tumor.

Microsurgical resections are frequently considered only for single metastases. Staged resections of multiple metastases via separate craniotomies have been described, but are not commonly performed (55). Small, isolated lesions deep to cortical surfaces may not be good candidates for resection because of difficulty with localization, despite advances in neurosurgical navigation technologies.

In contrast, radiosurgical treatment of multiple brain metastases can be performed in a single (usually outpatient) session, and the intracranial location of brain metastases usually does not present an issue for targeting in radiosurgery. An exception to this is for lesions located in close proximity to the optic chiasm. The limited tolerance of the optic nerves for single fraction treatment often compromises the ability to deliver radiosurgery to tumors juxtaposed with the optic apparatus (56). Fractionated treatment is an option for such metastases (57). Lesions selected for radiosurgical treatment are more likely to be controlled if they are small in size (41). Larger lesions are often treated with lower doses because of concern about injury to normal brain tissue from the larger scattered dose consequent to treating larger lesions (10). Neurosurgical resection of a large metastasis will provide a significant benefit from relief of mass effect.

## Stereotactic Radiosurgery Alone

Stereotactic radiosurgery alone as a primary treatment for metastatic disease has been performed, and good data regarding this approach has been published. In 1994, Flickinger et al. published a report on 116 patients from multiple institutions who had undergone radiosurgery alone or together with WBRT for solitary brain metastases (50). Median survival was 11 months after radiosurgery and 20 months after diagnosis. Local tumor control was excellent (85 percent of all patients followed), and radiation necrosis without viable tumor present was rare (1 percent). Two-year actuarial local tumor control rate was 67 percent ± 8 percent. Nine percent of patients required subsequent surgery for hemorrhage, necrosis, or tumor recurrence.

Sneed et al., in a 1999 review of 105 patients treated at the University of California at San Francisco (UCSF), observed no improvement in survival and local control with the addition of WBRT to SRS when salvage therapy was used for recurrence after SRS alone (58). However, prior to salvage, freedom from progression at 1 year was 28 percent for SRS alone versus 69 percent for WBRT + SRS. Moreover, for RPA Class I, median survival time was 35.3 months for RS alone and 12.9 months for RS + WBRT.

A further report by Sneed et al. in a 2002 multiinstitutional review found no improvement in overall survival when WBRT was added to SRS. Again, the RPA prognostic index was validated, though there was no improvement across the three classes with the addition of early whole-brain radiation to stereotactic radiosurgery. Overall survival was 14 versus 15.2, 8.2 versus 7, and 5.3 versus 5.5 months for SRS alone versus SRS + WBRT for RPA Class I, II, and III patients (59).

In the same year, a single-institution prospective study was reported by Regine et al., focusing on treating newly diagnosed brain metastases with SRS alone followed by observation (60). Median survival was 9 months. Brain tumor recurrence at the original site affected only 8 of 36 patients, and tumors recurred at both original and distant CNS sites in 3 of 36 patients. Tumors at distant sites only were found in 6 of 36 patients. Importantly, 12 of 17 recurrences were symptomatic, and 10 of 17 recurrences were associated with a neurologic deficit. Only 2 of 36 patients experienced RTOG Grade 3 or 4 toxicity attributable to SRS, and there were no deaths associated with SRS.

Varlotto et al. looked retrospectively at 110 patients who had received initial management with SRS with or without subsequent WBRT and had survived at least a year (61). Local control was improved with the addition of WBRT in patient with small tumor volume (<2 cm), single metastases, and lung cancer primary tumors in these relatively long surviving patients. There was no additional survival benefit with the addition of WBRT.

The best data available on anticipated outcomes for patients treated with stereotactic radiosurgery without early WBRT comes from a phase III trial reported by Aoyama et al. in 2006 (62). This Japanese trial involved 132 patients and randomized patients to SRS versus SRS+WBRT. Up to 4 brain metastases, each less than 3 cm, were allowed. Median survival was not significantly changed by the addition of WBRT (SRS + WBRT 7.5 months versus SRS alone 8 months, p=0.42). There were no significant differences in systemic and neurologic functional preservation or in toxic effects of radiation. Intracranial relapse did occur considerably more frequently in those patients who did not receive WBRT. Salvage treatment was frequently required when up-front WBRT was not used. The authors commented on a trend toward improved survival with the addition of WBRT, and a lack of incremental toxicity. However, improved intracranial control did not translate to a decrease in neurologic deaths. Importantly, follow-up imaging detected early recurrences before they became neurologically evident during clinical exam and KPS assessment by the clinician, and so this may have improved salvage treatment. Minimental state examination (MMSE) was optionally performed on some of the patients in the trial and showed there was no significant difference between the two arms.

The evidence shows that SRS is a safe treatment with low toxicity. CNS recurrence is more frequent with the omission of WBRT after SRS. With frequent imaging (62)—MRI scan 1–3 months after treatment, and every 3 months thereafter—there does not appear to be an effect on survival with the omission of WBRT, though this remains the subject of continued study in an ongoing randomized Intergroup trial (N0574) led by the North Central Cancer

Treatment Group (NCCTG) (63). This trial is also collecting neurocognitive testing data that will help evaluate endpoints other than survival in the study cohorts (63).

## Stereotactic Radiosurgery and Whole-Brain Radiation

While stereotactic radiosurgery is very effective at controlling oligometastases, intracranial control is compromised by the focal nature of this radiation technique. WBRT has been conventionally used prior to stereotactic radiosurgery as it is able to address the micrometastatic disease that is presumed to be present, is able to cytoreduce the radiographically evident metastatic deposits, and is also very easy to initiate in every radiation therapy department. In a meta-analysis of published stereotactic radiosurgery series, an improvement in overall survival was shown in comparison to historical controls for patients who underwent SRS in addition to WBRT. For RTOG RPA classes I, II, and III (discussed in the previous chapter), stereotactic radiosurgery with WBRT improved median survival to 16.1, 10.3, and 8.7 months versus 7.1, 4.2, 2.3 months for historical controls for WBRT alone. Also found to be statistically important was a controlled primary tumor, absence of extracranial disease, and higher Karnofsky performance status. Improvement in survival did not appear to be restricted by class for well-selected patients. This was obviously not a randomized population, and the influence on survival of the number of metastases was not discussed (64).

Patients included in retrospective series reporting the results from stereotactic radiosurgery have typically better results than patients who were not considered for stereotactic radiosurgery (33,65). Retrospective reports of stereotactic radiosurgery for brain metastases have reported an approximate 85 percent local control rate and a median survival of 9.4–11 months (32,50,65).

The RTOG performed a large randomized trial of 333 patients (RTOG 9508) that randomized RPA Class I and II patients to WBRT + SRS versus WBRT. Patients were enrolled who had KPS >70, and 1 to 3 metastases. WBRT in the trial was 2.5 Gy × 15 fractions for a total of 37.5 Gy over 3 weeks. Mets <2 cm in broadest diameter (in accordance with RTOG 90-05) were treated with a surface isodose of 24 Gy. Mets >2 cm but <3 cm were treated with 18 Gy, and those mets >3 cm and <4 cm were treated with 15 Gy. This study showed a survival benefit for SRS + WBRT versus WBRT alone (6.5 versus 4.9

months, p=0.0393) only for patients with a single metastasis (66). There was no survival benefit for the addition of SRS to WBRT for patients with more than one metastasis. On central review, local control was improved at 3 months and 1 year and there was a statistically significant improvement in functional status (as measured by KPS) and decreased steroid use at 6 months, though no difference in mental status was noted between the groups. There was no increased toxicity in the group that received SRS.

Interestingly, Kondziolka et al. performed a similar trial, which was closed after an interim analysis with only 27 patients randomized because of a very high local failure rate in the WBRT-alone arm versus the SRS + WBRT arm (100 percent versus 8 percent at 1 year). Patients were treated with 30 Gy in 12 fractions of 2.5 Gy. There was no significant improvement in overall survival benefit (11 versus 7.5 months) with this small sample size, but there was a 6-fold increase in local intracranial control of 36 months versus 6 months in favor of the SRS + WBRT arm. There was no neurologic or systemic morbidity related to stereotactic radiosurgery (67).

In a study that was published in abstract only, Chougule et al. randomized 96 patients to three separate arms: SRS alone, WBRT alone, or SRS + WBRT (68). Local control was improved for the SRS alone and SRS + WBRT arms compared to the WBRT alone arm (87 percent and 91 percent versus 62 percent), whereas median survival was highest for the WBRT alone arm (7 and 5 months versus 9 months). This trial did not include a control for whether patients had a surgical resection, and the number of patients enrolled may have been too small to demonstrate a survival benefit.

As noted in the previous section, Aoyama et al. performed a randomized controlled trial comparing SRS to SRS + WBRT. There was a significant improvement in prevention of brain tumor recurrence and intracranial relapse with the addition of WBRT (62).A survival benefit was not shown.

Selection of patients for treatment with stereotactic radiosurgery remains an area of continued study. Younger patients, well performing patients (KPS >70), and patients with 1 to 3 brain metastases are usually the patients selected for treatment, as the phase III RTOG 9508 trial appears to show improved outcomes in terms of overall survival, metastasis control, and steroid usage with the addition of SRS to WBRT for these selected patients (66). In addition, the number of metastases treated by SRS may influence whether a patient benefits. Well performing (KPS>70) patients with two or solitary metastases have a much improved survival time in comparison to patients with three or more metastases: 211+ weeks versus 63 weeks, p=<0.002 (69). For patients with four or more metastases, it is unclear whether there is a benefit to radiosurgery in addition to WBRT. Some authors have retrospectively observed an improvement in overall survival (70,71), whereas others have observed improvement only for young patients (<45 years) (72). At present, the use of SRS with WBRT may be considered a very reasonable option for well performing patients or young patients with a limited volume or number of metastases (73).

In summary, no randomized trial has shown a survival benefit for the addition of WBRT to SRS, however there is evidence for improved local control and reduction in time until salvage therapy is necessary. Conversely, there does not seem to be significant additional toxicity with the addition of SRS to WBRT. In patients with oligometastases (2–4), the use of SRS before or after WBRT is reasonable in highly functioning patients [KPS >70] (73). WBRT may also be delayed until recurrence without a detriment to overall survival. For single metastases that are not surgically accessible, Class I data shows that SRS + WBRT is preferable to WBRT (66). SRS alone may be given versus SRS + WBRT with the knowledge that frequent MRI imaging follow up is necessary, and salvage therapy is more often needed and may be required sooner if WBRT is omitted.

## Prophylactic Cranial Irradiation

Whole-brain radiation is also used as prophylaxis in prevention of brain metastases for cancers with a predilection for spread to or within the CNS, including medulloblastoma as a part of craniospinal irradiation (74), very high risk acute lymphocytic leukemia (75), and small cell lung cancer (76–82).

When prophylactic cranial irradiation (PCI) is used in the setting of small cell lung cancer (SCLC) in complete remission, the median duration of survival increases from 12 to 20 months (82), with reports of 4-year survival around 22 percent [95 percent CI: 15–32 percent] (76). Thus, it appears that for selected small cell lung cancer patients, survival after whole-brain radiation therapy can be extended by over a year or more. In addition, a meta-analysis of all English and French language randomized trials regarding PCI in small cell lung cancer patients published before January 2000, has confirmed a survival benefit in patients in clinical remission, with a hazard ratio (HR) for death of 0.82 [95 percent CI : 0.71–0.96] (83).

PCI for patients with extensive stage small cell lung cancer who have partial or complete response to treatment has also recently been shown to infer a survival benefit (27.1 percent versus 13.3 percent 1-year overall survival, p=0.0033). The risk of symptomatic brain metastases was significantly reduced, with a 1-year cumulative incidence of symptomatic brain metastases of 14.6 percent on PCI versus 40.4 for controls [p<0.0001] (84).

Typical doses for PCI for SCLC are lower than for definitive or adjuvant WBRT for existing metastases. A commonly used dose is 36 Gy in 18 fractions, or 30 Gy in 15 fractions, and is applied in similar approach to that used in WBRT for existing metastases, using a helmet field technique (83). The European Organization for Research and Treatment of Cancer (EORTC) extensive stage PCI trial uses doses ranging from 20 Gy in 5 fractions of 4 Gy to 30 Gy in 10 fractions of 3 Gy (84). Other trials have recommended 24–30 Gy in 3 Gy fractions or less (76). Multiple studies have looked into neurocognitive sequelae from PCI and whether these outweigh the benefit seen in survival. Current National Comprehensive Cancer Network (NCCN) guidelines strongly support PCI in patients with limited disease with a complete response (Category 1 recommendation) and recommend treatment in patients with extensive disease with a complete response (Category 2B recommendation) (85). A recent EORTC trial reported the results of a randomized trial of PCI versus no PCI in 286 patients with extensive disease small cell lung cancer after any response to chemotherapy. PCI significantly reduced the risk of symptomatic brain metastases (14.6 percent versus 40.4 percent at 1 year, p<0.0001) and improved both progression-free survival and overall survival (27.1 percent versus 13.3 percent at 1 year, p=0.0033) (84). This strongly suggests that PCI can now be considered in all extensive disease patients who show a response to chemotherapy to reduce the incidence of symptomatic brain metastases and prolong disease-free and overall survival (86).

There does appear to be a radiation dose response relationship in reduction of brain metastases in PCI, with doses approximating 36 Gy in 18 fractions effective compared to lower doses without a significant increase in neurocognitive deficit (80,82). There has not been a survival benefit accredited to higher doses. Other investigators have found a lower dose response threshold of 25.2 Gy in reducing brain metastasis risk (87).

Twice daily fractionation for PCI has also been investigated in an attempt to reduce late neurotoxicity (88). This trial treated patients to 30–36 Gy in twice daily fractions of 1.5 Gy and was well tolerated. This treatment regimen is under further investigation (RTOG 0212) (89).

# Future Directions and Areas of Investigation

## Concurrent Chemotherapy with WBRT

Multiple studies have attempted to improve the efficacy of whole-brain radiation with the use of radiosensitizing cytotoxic chemotherapeutic agents. These studies have been largely disappointing with no benefit in terms of median survival or objective response rates.

Guerreri et al. tested at concomitant carboplatin and whole-brain radiation for brain metastases from non-small cell lung cancer, but the study did not show a benefit in terms of objective response or survival (90). Other investigators have also looked at various combinations of chemotherapy (carboplatin, ifosfamide, and vinorelbine-ifosfamide-cisplatin) with whole-brain radiation and have noted similar side effects without the expected severe neurotoxicity, and with good response rates (91–93), but this approach remains highly experimental. The most frequent acute complication seems to be myelosuppression from the concurrent chemotherapies used.

Use of the potent radiosensitizer gemcitabine and WBRT has been investigated in a phase I trial escalating the dose of twice-weekly gemcitabine. At higher dose levels, 2 toxic deaths were encountered. A small number of patients have been treated, and so a maximum tolerated dose (MTD) of gemcitabine given twice weekly was defined as 62.5 mg/m$^2$ (94). A phase II study of gemcitabine given twice weekly at the dose of 50.0 mg/m$^2$ is underway in the United Kingdom (UK).

Topotecan, which has shown promising efficacy in patients with heavily pretreated SCLC brain metastases (95), has also been investigated in conjunction with WBRT in a phase I/II trial. Maximum tolerated dose was $12 \times 0.5$ mg/m$^2$ in chemotherapy naive patients and $12 \times 0.4$ mg/m$^2$ in chemo-pretreated patients (96). A phase III study is now underway.

Two groups, Antonadou et al. (97) and Verger et al. (98) have performed randomized phase II trials evaluating neurotoxicity in patients with brain metastases randomized to WBRT versus temozolamide + WBRT. Both trials found statistically significant improvement in intracranial control and response with the addition of temozolamide to radiotherapy. As expected, there was worsened hematologic toxicity and nausea and vomiting in patients receiving temozolamide, but this was readily managed with supportive measures. There seemed to be an improvement in neurologic response to treatment, and less steroid use and a lower death rate from brain metastases progression. Again, this approach remains experimental and is the subject of further investigation.

Novel and traditional systemic anticancer therapy with or without WBRT continues to be an area of investigation (73), with phase III trials involving the combination of radiation and temozolomide with erlotinib (99) and oral topotecan (100) underway.

## Radiation Sensitizing Agents

Unfortunately, all trials of radiation sensitizing agents without intrinsic antitumor effects have been negative. There have been several large clinical trials mounted recently evaluating the use of agents with promising preclinical profiles, but these were unfortunately also negative. There is, however, still some hope for this approach in managing brain metastases.

Motexafin gadolinium (gadolinium texaphyrin, MGd) is a porphyrin-like paramagnetic molecule that disrupts redox-dependent pathways in cells, inhibits oxidative stress-related proteins, and induces apoptosis. In preclinical trials, it was shown to enhance radiation sensitivity in cells that take up the drug (101). Interestingly, MGd has been shown to localize within tumors, and because of its paramagnetic nature, can demonstrate brain metastases on noncontrast MRI (102). A phase III randomized trial of 401 patients was mounted to evaluate the efficacy of WBRT with or without concurrent MGd (103). This trial was also important in its careful neurocognitive testing of all patients, allowing for one of the most thorough examinations of acute and chronic neurologic sequelae from WBRT.

Unfortunately, there was no improvement in median overall survival between the two arms (5.2 months for MGd + WBRT versus 4.9 months for WBRT alone, p=0.48). There was also no difference between the two arms in terms of median time to neurologic progression (9.5 months for MGd + WBRT versus 8.3 months for WBRT, p=0.95).

In unplanned subset analyses of the above trial, the time to overall neurologic progression in non-small cell lung cancer patients (n=251) was significantly increased (median not reached for MGd + WBRT versus 7.4 months for WBRT; p=0.048) (104). Therefore, a confirmatory phase III trial was performed for this subset of patients with non-small cell cancer (NSCLC) brain metastases. Five hundred fifty-four patients with NSCLC brain metastases and KPS >70 were randomized to WBRT + MGd versus WBRT alone.

Unfortunately, this too was a negative trial, as time to overall neurologic progression between the two arms was not significantly different: WBRT + MGd 15.4 months versus WBRT alone 10 months (104). There was a 6.4 month difference in the median time to neurologic progression in the 805 NSCLC patients enrolled on these two phase III studies that received MGd and WBRT compared to WBRT alone: p = 0.016 (105). An application to the FDA for the use of MGd with radiation therapy for NSCLC brain metastases was not successful (http://www.pharmacyclics.com/wt/page/xcytrin).

Importantly, the MGd trial shed some light on the pretreatment neurocognitive function of patients with brain metastases who undergo WBRT. Ninety-five percent of patients had impairment of one or more neurocognitive tests at baseline, and 42.4 percent of patients had impairment in 4 or more tests (out of 7), indicating severe neurocognitive dysfunction (106). Patients with a greater total volume of lesions had worsened neurocognitive function, whereas the overall number of lesions was not statistically correlated with baseline neurocognitive function. Baseline neurocognitive function was predictive of overall survival. The authors noted that a combination of neurocognitive testing and tumor prognostic variables predicted survival better than tumor variables alone.

Efaproxiral (Efaproxyn, RSR13; Allos Therapeutics Inc., Westminster, CO) is a pharmaceutical agent that reduces the oxygen-binding affinity of hemoglobin, facilitating the release of oxygen in hypoxic regions (107). It was theorized that efaproxiral could increase the effectiveness of WBRT by improving the radiosensitivity of the hypoxic fraction of brain metastases. Although the phase III trial that was mounted to investigate the use of efaproxiral in conjunction with WBRT was negative overall, there appeared to be a subset of breast cancer patients who had derived a survival benefit from efaproxiral (108). Unfortunately, the confirmatory phase III trial for this subset of patients was also negative for the primary endpoints of survival and response to treatment (109).

## Improvement in Radiation Delivery

Intensity modulated radiation therapy (IMRT) is a radiation delivery technique that allows for improved dose distributions by varying the intensity of radiation delivered within different parts of a radiation field. The improved ability to distribute radiation dose has been used to decreased the dose delivered to the scalp in an attempt to reduce treatment associated alopecia (110), and

IMRT has also been used to improve dose homogeneity in WBRT (111), although clinical trials comparing IMRT to conventional delivery techniques have not been mounted.

IMRT has also been investigated as a means to spare the hippocampus of the brain from radiation. Radiation induced neurotoxicity involves functions that are associated with the hippocampus, including memory, learning, and spatial information processing (112). Animal studies suggest that even low doses of radiation (2 Gy) can cause damage to the hippocampus (113). Studies investigating the use of conformal radiation techniques to avoid the hippocampus while treating the rest of the brain are underway. Retrospective review of patterns of brain metastasis shows that only 3.3 percent of all brain metastases occur within the hippocampus and a 5 mm margin. Eight percent of all patients (95 percent CI 3.5–15.2 percent) developed a brain metastasis within a 5 mm margin of the hippocampus (114,115). Investigators argue that radiosurgery could readily be used as salvage therapy for any patients who develop brain metastases in the hippocampus after hippocampus-sparing WBRT.

Image guided radiation therapy (IGRT), which involves daily pretreatment verification of the accuracy of targeting, has been used to deliver higher daily doses to metastases more precisely while delivering conventional doses to the rest of the brain (116). The role of IMRT and IGRT in the treatment of brain metastases is still being investigated, and potential benefits to patients from these more sophisticated therapies remains to be proven.

The use of SRS instead of WBRT after surgical resection has also been investigated, and the crude local control rate (14 percent) at a median follow up of 14.8 months (range 2.0–80.0 months) appears equivalent to WBRT. Actuarial local control at 1 year was 79 percent. Investigators targeted the resection cavity and a 0–2 mm margin for SRS. Theoretically, this technique could avoid the side effects of irradiation of normal brain; because it is a focal therapy, it will not affect the risk of intracranial recurrence elsewhere in the brain (117). More investigation with longer follow up and toxicity metrics is necessary before this becomes routine clinical practice.

## Prophylactic Cranial Irradiation for Other Histologies

Long-surviving patients with advanced or metastatic HER2+ breast carcinoma treated with trastuzumab (Herceptin) have a high rate of metastatic brain disease: 21 percent in one retrospective series (118). Because of this, a clinical trial of prophylactic cranial irradiation has been suggested as reasonable (119). In addition, lapatinib (Tykerb), an oral small molecule inhibitor of the tyrosine kinase activity of epidermal growth factor receptor (EGFR) and HER-2, is being investigated in the setting of trastuzumab refractory HER2+ breast cancer metastatic to the brain (120). Lapatinib is a smaller molecule than trastuzumab and is suspected to be more capable of crossing the blood-brain barrier; it has been shown to have activity in brain metastases regrowing after WBRT (121). Investigation of lapatinib in combination with WBRT ± SRS for established metastatic disease is ongoing (122).

Several randomized and nonrandomized trials have investigated the efficacy of prophylactic whole-brain radiation therapy in non-small cell lung cancer (123–126). Although no survival benefit has been shown in these trials individually, there is evidence of a reduction in the absolute incidence of brain metastases (127). The RTOG is currently sponsoring an ongoing phase III prospective randomized trial investigating the overall survival benefit from the use of prophylactic cranial irradiation in non-small cell lung cancer (RTOG 0214) (128).

## References

1. Posner JB, Chernik NL. Intracranial metastases from systemic cancer. *Adv Neurol* 1978;19:579–592.
2. Posner JB. Management of brain metastases. *Rev Neurol* 1992;148:477–482.
3. Delattre JY, Krol G, Thaler HT, et al. Distribution of brain metastases. *Arch Neurol* 1988;45:741–744.
4. Bouffet E, Doumi N. Brain metastases in children with solid tumors. *Cancer* 1997;79; 403–410.
5. Tasdemiroglu E, Patchell RA. Cerebral metastases in childhood malignancies. *Acta Neurochir (Wien)* 1997;139:182–187.
6. Johnson JD, Young B. Demographics of brain metastasis. *Neurosurg Clin North Am* 1996;7:337–344.
7. Lassman AB, DeAngelis LM. Brain metastases. *Neurol Clin* 2003;21:1–23,vii.
8. Coia LR. The role of radiation therapy in the treatment of brain metastases. *Int J Radiat Oncol Biol Phys* 1992;23:229–238.
9. Barnholtz-Sloan JS, Sloan AE, Davis FG, et al. Incidence proportions of brain metastases in patients diagnosed (1973 to 2001) in the Metropolitan Detroit Cancer Surveillance System. *J Clin Oncol* 2004;22:2865–2867.
10. Cairncross JG, Kim JH, Posner JB. Radiation therapy for brain metastases. *Ann Neurol* 1980;7:529–541.
11. Chambers A, Groom A, MacDonald I. Dissemination and growth of cancer cells in metastatic sites. *Nat Cancer Rev* 2002;2:563–572.
12. Steeg PS. Tumor metastasis: mechanistic insights and clinical challenges. *Nat Med* 2006; 12:895–904.
13. Hwang TL, Close TP, Grego JM, et al. Predilection of brain metastasis in gray and white matter junction and vascular border zones. *Cancer* 1996;77: 1551–1555.

14. Nussbaum ES, Djalilian HR, Cho KH. Brain metastases. Histology, multiplicity, surgery, and survival. *Cancer* 1996;78:1781–1793.
15. Schellinger PD, Meinck HM, Thron A. Diagnostic accuracy of MRI compared to CT in patients with brain metastases. *J Neurooncol* 1999;44:275–281.
16. Davis PC, Hudgins PA, Peterman SB, Hoffman JC. Diagnosis of cerebral metastases: Double-dose delayed CT versus contrast-enhanced MR imaging. *Am J Neuroradiol* 1991;12:293–300.
17. Runge VM, Kirsh JE, Burke VJ, et al. High dose gadoteridol in MR imaging of intracranial neoplasms. *J Magn Reson Imaging* 1992;2:9–18.
18. Sze G, Milano E, Johnson C, et al. Detection of brain metastases: Comparison of contrast-enhanced MR with unenhanced MR and enhanced CT. *Am J Neuroradiol* 1990;11:785–791.
19. Schneider G, Kirchin MA, Pirovano G, et al. Gadobenate dimeglumine-enhanced magnetic resonance imaging of intracranial metastases: Effect of dose on lesion detection and delineation. *J Magn Reson Imaging* 2001;14:525–539.
20. Kuhn MJ, Hammer GM, Swenson LC, et al. MRI evaluation of "solitary" brain metastases with triple-dose gadoteridol: Comparison with contrast-enhanced CT and conventional-dose gadopentetate dimeglumine MRI studies in the same patients. *Comput Med Imaging Graph* 1994;18:391–399.
21. Engh JA, Flickinger JC, Niranjan A, et al. Optimizing intracranial metastasis detection for stereotactic radiosurgery. *Stereotact Funct Neurosurg* 2007;85: 162–168.
22. Ruderman NB, Hall TC. Use of glucocorticoids in the palliative treatment of metastatic brain tumors. *Cancer* 1965;18:298–306.
23. Stuschke M, Eberhardt W, Pottgen C, et al. Prophylactic cranial irradiation in locally advanced non-small-cell lung cancer after multimodality treatment: long-term follow-up and investigations of late neuropsychologic effects. *J Clin Oncol* 1999;17:2700–2709.
24. DeAngelis LM, Delattre JY, Posner JB. Radiation-induced dementia in patients cured of brain metastases. *Neurology* 1989;39:789–796.
25. Klein M, Heimans JJ, Aaronson NK, et al. Effect of radiotherapy and other treatment-related factors on mid-term to long-term cognitive sequelae in low-grade gliomas: A comparative study. *Lancet* 2002;360:1361–1368.
26. Coia LR. The role of radiation therapy in the treatment of brain metastases. *Int J Radiat Oncol Biol Phys* 1993;23:229–237.
27. Komarnicky LT, Phillips TL, Martz K, et al. A randomized phase III protocol for the evaluation of misonidazole combined with radiation in the treatment of patients with brain metastases (RTOG 79-16). *Int J Radiat Oncol Biol Phys* 1991;20:53–58.
28. Sause WT, Crowley JJ, Morantz R, et al. Solitary brain metastases: Results of an RTOG/SWOG protocol evaluating surgery + RT versus RT alone. *Am J Clin Oncol* 1990; 13:427–432.
29. Langer CJ, Mehta MP. Current management of brain metastases, with a focus on systemic options. *J Clin Oncol* 2005;23:6207–6219.
30. Mehta MP, Khuntia D. Current strategies in whole-brain radiation therapy for brain metastases. *Neurosurgery* 2005;57(Suppl):S4–33.
31. Thames HD, Withers HR, Peters LH, et al. Changes in early and late radiation responses with altered dose fractionation: Implications for dose-survival relationships. *Int J Radiat Oncol Biol Phys* 1982;8:219–226.
32. Muacevic A, Kreth FW, Mack A, et al. Stereotactic radiosurgery without radiation therapy providing high local tumor control of multiple brain metastases from renal cell carcinoma. *Minim Invas Neurosurg* 2004;47:203–208.
33. Samlowski WE, Watson GA, Wang M, et al. Multimodality treatment of melanoma brain metastases incorporating stereotactic radiosurgery (SRS). *Cancer* 2007; Epub 9 March 2007.
34. Koc M, McGregor J, Grecula J, et al. Gamma Knife radiosurgery for intracranial metastatic melanoma: An analysis of survival and prognostic factors. *J Neurooncol* 2005;71: 307–313.

35. Hoshi S, Jokura H, Nakamura H, et al. Gamma-knife radiosurgery for brain metastasis of renal cell carcinoma: Results in 42 patients. *Int J Urol* 2002;9: 618–625.

36. Berk L. An overview of radiotherapy trials for the treatment of brain metastases. *Oncology (Williston Park)* 1995;9:1205–1212.

37. Order SE, Hellman S, Von Essen CF, et al. Improvement in quality of survival following whole-brain irradiation for brain metastases. *Radiology* 1968;91:149–153.

38. Gaspar L, Scott C, Rotman M, et al. Recursive partitioning analysis (RPA) of prognostic factors in three Radiation Therapy Oncology Group (RTOG) brain metastases trials. *Int J Radiat Oncol Biol Phys* 1997;37:745–751.

39. Borgelt B, Gelber R, Kramer S, et al. The palliation of brain metastases: Final results of the first two studies by the Radiation Therapy Oncology Group. *Int J Radiat Oncol Biol Phys* 1980;6:1–9.

40. Vogelbaum MA, Suh JH. Resectable brain metastases. *J Clin Oncol* 2006;24:1289–1294.

41. Mehta M, Noyes W, Craig B, et al. A cost-effectiveness and cost-utility analysis of radiosurgery versus resection for single-brain metastases. *Int J Radiat Oncol Biol Phys* 1997;39: 445–454.

42. Patchell RA, Tibbs PA, Walsh JW, et al. A randomized trial of surgery in the treatment of single metastases. *N Engl J Med* 1990;322:494–500.

43. Vecht CJ, Haaxma-Reiche H, Noordijk EM, et al. Treatment of single brain metastases: Radiotherapy alone or combined with neurosurgery? *Ann Neurol* 1993;33:583–590.

44. Mintz AP, Kestle J, Rathbone MP, et al. A randomized trial to assess the efficacy of surgery in addition to radiotherapy in patients with a single brain metastasis. *Cancer* 1996; 78:1470–1476.

45. Noordijk EM, Vecht CJ, Haaxma-Reiche H. The choice of treatment of single brain metastasis should be based on extracranial tumor activity and age. *Int J Radiat Oncol Biol Phys* 1994;29:711–717.

46. DeAngelis LM, Mandell LR, Thaler HT, et al. The role of postoperative radiotherapy after resection of single brain metastases. *Neurosurgery.* 1989;24: 798–805.

47. Dosoretz DE, Blitzer PH, Russell AH, et al. Management of solitary metastases to the brain: The role of elective brain irradiation following complete surgical resection. *Int J Radiat Oncol Biol Phys* 1980;6:1727–1730.

48. Patchell RA, Ribbs PA, Regine WF, et al. Postoperative Radiotherapy in the Treatment of Single Metastases to the Brain. *JAMA* 1998;280:1485–1489.

49. Rutigliano MJ, Lunsford LD, Kondziolka D, et al. The cost effectiveness of stereotactic radiosurgery versus surgical resection in the treatment of solitary metastatic brain tumors. *Neurosurgery* 1995;37:445–453.

50. Flickinger JC, Kondziolka D, Lunsford LD, et al. A multi-institutional experience with stereotactic radiosurgery for solitary brain metastasis. *Int J Radiat Oncol Biol Phys* 1994; 28:797–802.

51. Mehta MP, Rozental JM, Levin AB, et al. Defining the role of radiosurgery in the management of brain metastases. *Int J Radiat Oncol Biol Phys* 1992;24:619–625.

52. Shaw E, Scott C, Souhami L, et al. Single dose radiosurgical treatment of recurrent previously irradiated primary brain tumors and brain metastases. *Int J Radiat Oncol Biol Phys* 2000;47:269–271.

53. Shehata MK, Young AB, Reid B, et al. Stereotactic radiosurgery (SRS) of 468 brain metastases 2 cm: Implications for SRS dose and whole brain radiation therapy (WBRT). *Int J Radiat Oncol Biol Phys* 2002;54(Suppl);94.[Abstract].

54. Muacevic A, Kreth FW, Horstmann GA, et al. Surgery and radiotherapy compared with Gamma Knife radiosurgery in the treatment of solitary cerebral metastases of small diameter. *J Neurosurg* 1999;91:35–43

55. Bindal RK, Sawaya R, Leavens ME, et al. Surgical treatment of multiple brain metastases. *J Neurosurg* 1993;79:210–216.

56. Tishler RB, Loeffler JS, Lunsford LD, et al. Tolerance of cranial nerves of the cavernous sinus to radiosurgery. *Int J Radiat Oncol Biol Phys* 1993;27:215–221.

57. Pham CJ, Chang SD, Gibbs IC, et al. Preliminary visual field preservation after staged CyberKnife radiosurgery for perioptic lesions. *Neurosurgery* 2004;54: 799–810.

58. Sneed PK, Lamborn KR, Forstner JM, et al. Radiosurgery for Brain Metastases: Is Whole Brain Radiotherapy Necessary? *Int J Radiat Oncol Biol Phys* 1999;43: 549–558.

59. Sneed PK, Suh JH, Goetsch SJ. A multi-institutional review of radiosurgery alone versus radiosurgery with whole brain radiotherapy as the initial management of brain metastases. *Int J Radiat Oncol Biol Phys* 2002;54:519–526.

60. Regine WF, Huhn JL, Patchell RA, et al. Risk of symptomatic brain tumor recurrence and neurologic deficit after radiosurgery alone in patients with newly diagnosed brain metastases: Results and implications. *Int J Radiat Oncol Biol Phys* 2002;52:333–338.

61. Varlotto JM, Flickinger JC, Niranjan A, et al. The impact of whole-brain radiation therapy on long-term control and morbidity of patients surviving more than one year after Gamma Knife radiosurgery for brain metastases. *Int J Radiat Oncol Biol Phys* 2005;62: 1125–1132.

62. Aoyama H, Shirato H, Tago M, et al. Stereotactic radiosurgery plus whole-brain radiation therapy versus stereotactic radiosurgery alone for treatment of brain metastasis: A randomized controlled trial. *JAMA* 2006;295:2483–2491.

63. Phase III randomized study of stereotactic radiosurgery with versus without whole-brain radiotherapy in patients with cerebral metastases. Available at: http://www.cancer.gov/clinicaltrials/NCCTG-N0574. Accessed July 1, 2007.

64. Sanghavi SN, Miranpuri SS, Chappell R, et al. Radiosurgery for patients with brain metastases: A multi-institutional analysis, stratified by the RTOG recursive partitioning analysis method. *Int J Radiat Oncol Biol Phys* 2001;51:426–434.

65. Alexander E, Moriarty TM, Davis RB, et al. Stereotactic radiosurgery for the definitive, non-invasive treatment of brain metastases. *J Natl Cancer Inst* 1995;87:34–40.

66. Andrews DW, Scott CB, Sperduto PW, et al. Whole brain radiation therapy with or without stereotactic radiosurgery boost for patients with one to three brain metastases: phase III results of the RTOG 9508 randomised trial. *Lancet* 2004; 363:1665–1672.

67. Kondziolka D, Patel A, Lunsford LD, et al. Stereotactic radiosurgery plus whole brain radiotherapy versus radiotherapy alone for patients with multiple brain metastases. *Int J Radiat Oncol Biol Phys* 1999;45;427–434.

68. Chougule PB, Burton-Williams M, Saris S, et al. Randomized treatment of brain metastasis with Gamma Knife radiosurgery, whole brain radiotherapy, or both. *Int J Radiat Oncol Biol Phys* 2000;48(Suppl):114[Abstract].

69. Joseph J, Adler JR, Cox RS, et al. Linear accelerator-based stereotaxic radiosurgery for brain metastases: the influence of number of lesions on survival. *J Clin Oncol* 1996;14: 1085–1092.

70. Nam TK, Lee JI, Jung YJ, et al. Gamma Knife surgery for brain metastases in patients harboring four or more lesions: survival and prognostic factors. *J Neurosurg* 2005;(102 Suppl):147–150.

71. Bhatnagar, AK, Flickinger JC, Kondziolka D, et al. Stereotactic radiosurgery for four or more intracranial metastases. *Int J Radiat Oncol Biol Phys* 2006;64: 898–903.

72. Diluna ML, King JT, Knisely JP, et al. Prognostic factors for survival after stereotactic radiosurgery vary with the number of cerebral metastases. *Cancer* 2007;109:135–145.

73. Rao RD, Brown PD, Buckner JC. Innovation in the management of brain metastases. *Oncology (Williston Park)* 2007;21:473–481.

74. Packer RJ, Goldwein J, Nicholson HS, et al. Treatment of children with medulloblastomas with reduced-dose craniospinal radiation therapy and adjuvant chemotherapy: A Children's Cancer Group study. *J Clin Onc* 1999;17: 2127–2136.

75. Pui CH, Evans WE, Treatment of acute lymphoblastic leukemia. *N Engl J Med* 2006; 354:166–178.

76. Laplanche A, Monnet I, Santos-Miranda JA, et al. Controlled clinical trial of prophylactic cranial irradiation for patients with small-cell lung cancer in complete remission. *Lung Cancer* 1998; 21:193–201.

77. Jackson DV, Richards F, Cooper R, et al. Prophylactic cranial irradiation in small cell carcinoma of the lung. *JAMA* 1977;237:2730–2733.

78. Maurer LH, Tulloh M, Weiss RB, et al. A randomized combined modality trial in small cell carcinoma of the lung. *Cancer* 1980;45:30–39.

79. Arriagada R, Le Chevalier T, Boire F, et al. Prophylactic cranial irradiation for patients with small-cell lung cancer in complete remission. *J Natl Cancer Inst* 1995;87: 183–190.

80. Gregor A, Cull A, Stephens RJ, et al. Prophylactic cranial irradiation is indicated following complete response to induction therapy in small cell lung cancer: results of multicentre randomized trial. *Eur J Cancer* 1997;33:1752–1758.

81. Shaw EG, Su JQ, Eagan RT, et al. Prophylactic cranial irradiation in complete responders with small-cell lung cancer: analysis of the Mayo Clinic and North Central Cancer Treatment Group databases. *J Clin Oncol* 1994;12:2327–2332.

82. Auperin A, Arriagada R, Pignon JP, et al. Prophylactic cranial irradiation For patients with small-cell lung cancer in complete remission. *N Eng J Med* 1999; 341:476–484.

83. Meert AP, Paesmans M, Berghmans T. Prophylactic cranial irradiation in small cell lung cancer: A systematic review of the literature with meta-analysis. *BMC Cancer* 2001;1:5.

84. Slotman B, Faivre-Finn C, Kramer G. Prophylactic cranial irradiation in extensive small-cell lung cancer. *N Engl J Med* 2007;357:664–72.

85. Johnson BE, Crawford J, Downey RJ, et al. Small cell lung cancer clinical practice guidelines in oncology. *J Natl Compr Canc Netw* 2006;6:602–622.

86. Castrucci, WA, Knisely JPS. An update on the treatment of CNS metastases in small cell lung cancer. *Canc J Sci Am* 2008. In press.

87. Rubenstein JH, Dosoretz DE, Katin MJ, et al. Low doses of prophylactic cranial irradiation effective in limited stage small cell carcinoma of the lung. *Int J Radiat Oncol Biol Phys* 1995;33:329–337.

88. Wolfson AH, Bains Y, Lu J, et al. Twice-daily prophylactic cranial irradiation for patients with limited disease small-cell lung cancer with complete response to chemotherapy and consolidative therapy. *Am J Clin Oncol (CCT)* 2001;24: 290–295.

89. Brain irradiation in treating patients with limited-stage small cell lung cancer. Available at: http://clinicaltrials.gov/show/NCT00057746. Accessed July 13, 2007.

90. Guerreri M, Wong K, Ryan G. A randomized phase III study of palliative radiation with concomitant carboplatin for brain metastases from non-small cell carcinoma of the lung. *Lung Cancer* 2004;46:107–111.

91. Quantin X, Khial F, Reme-Saumon M, et al. Concomitant brain radiotherapy and vinorelbine-ifosfamide-cisplatin chemotherapy in brain metastases of non-small cell lung cancer. *Lung Cancer* 1999;26:35–39.

92. Quantin X, Pujol JL, Paris A, et al. Concomitant brain radiotherapy and high-dose ifosfamide in brain relapses of lung cancer. *Ann Oncol* 1997;8:911–913.

93. Furuse K, Kamimori T, Kawahara M. A pilot study of concurrent whole-brain radiotherapy and chemotherapy combined with cisplatin, vindesine and mitomycin in non small cell lung cancer with brain metastasis. *Br J Cancer* 1997; 75:614–618.

94. Maraveyas A, Sgouros J, Upadhyay S, et al. Gemcitabine twice weekly as a radiosensitiser for the treatment of brain metastases in patients with carcinoma: a phase I study. *Br J Cancer* 2005;92:815–819.

95. Korfel A, Oehm C, Pawel JV, et al. Response to topotecan of symptomatic brain metastases of small-cell lung cancer also after whole-brain irradiation: A multicenter phase II study. *Eur J Cancer* 2002;38:1724–1729.

96. Kocher M, Eich HT, Semrau R, et al. Phase I/II trial of simultaneous whole-brain irradiation and dose-escalating topotecan for brain metastases. *Strahlenther Onkol* 2005;181:20–25.

97. Antonadou D, Paraskevaidis M, Sarris G, et al. Phase II randomized trial of temozolamide and concurrent radiotherapy in patients with brain metastases. *J Clin Oncol* 2002;20: 3644–3650.

98. Verger E, Gil M, Yaya R, et al. Temozolomide and concomitant whole brain radiotherapy in patients with brain metastases: A phase II randomized trial. *Int J Radiat Oncol Biol Phys* 2005;61:185–191.

99. Radiation therapy and stereotactic radiosurgery with or without temozolomide or erlotinib in treating patients with brain metastases secondary to non-small cell lung cancer. Available at: http://clinicaltrials.gov/show/NCT00096265. Accessed July 13, 2007.

100. Oral Hycamtin plus whole brain radiation therapy in treatment of brain metastases resulting from non-small lung cancer. Available at: http://clinicaltrials.gov/show/NCT00390806. Accessed July 13, 2007.

101. Rockwell S, Donnelly ET, Liu Y, et al. Preliminary studies of the effects of gadolinium texaphyrin on the growth and radiosensitivity of EMT6 cells in vitro. *Int J Radiat Oncol Biol Phys* 2002;54:536–541.

102. Viala J, Vanel D, Meingan P, et al. Phases IB and II multidose trial of gadolinium texaphrin, a radiation sensitizer detectable at MR imaging: Preliminary results in brain metastases. *Radiology* 1999;212:755–759.

103. Mehta MP, Rodrigus P, Terhaard CHJ, et al. Survival and neurologic outcomes in a randomized trial of motexafin gadolinium and whole brain radiation therapy in brain metastases. *J Clin Oncol* 2003;21:2529–2536.

104. Mehta M, Carrie C, Mahe MA, et al. Motexafin gadolinium (MGd) combined with prompt whole brain radiation therapy prolongs time to neurologic progression in non-small cell lung cancer (NSCLC) patients with brain metastases: Results of a randomized phase 3 trial. *Int J Radiat Oncol Biol Phys* 2006; 66(Suppl):S23[Abstract].

105. Pharmacyclics press release from April 23, 2007. Available at: http://ir.pharmacyclics.com/releases.cfm. Accessed 13 August 2007.

106. Meyers CA, Smith JA, Bezjak A, et al. Neurocognitive function and progression in patients with brain metastases treated with whole-brain radiation and motexafin gadolinium: results of a randomized phase III trial. *J Clin Oncol* 2004;22:157–165.

107. Charpentier MM. Efaproxiral: A radiation enhancer used in brain metastases from breast cancer. *Ann Pharmacother* 2005;39:2038–2045.

108. Suh JH, Baldassare S, Abdenour N, et al. Phase III Study of Efaproxiral as an adjunct to whole-brain radiation therapy for brain metastases. *J Clin Oncol* 2006;24:106–114.

109. Allos therapeutics reports results for phase 3 Enrich study of Efaproxyn in women with brain metastases originating from breast cancer. Available at: http://ir.allos.com/phoenix.zhtml?c=125475&p=irol-newsArticle&ID=1016824. Accessed July 13, 2007.

110. Roberge D, Parker W, Niazi TM, Olivares M. Treating the contents and not the container: Dosimetric study of hair-sparing whole brain intensity modulated radiation therapy. *Technol Cancer Res Treat* 2005;4:567–570.

111. Yu JB, Shiao SL, Knisely JPS. A dosimetric evaluation of conventional helmet field irradiation versus two-field intensity-modulated radiation therapy technique. *Int J Radiat Oncol Biol Phys* 2007;68:621–631.

112. Montje ML, Palmer T. Radiation injury and neurogenesis. *Curr Opin Neurol* 2003;16:129–134.

113. Van der Kogel AJ. Radiation-induced damage in the central nervous system: An interpretation of target cell responses. *Br J Cancer* 1986;7(Suppl):207–217.

114. Khuntia D, Brown P, Li J. Whole-brain radiotherapy in the management of brain metastases. *J Clin Oncol* 2006;24:1295–1304.

115. Ghia A, Tome AW, Thomas S, et al. Distribution of brain metastases in relation to the hippocampus: Implications for neurocognitive functional preservation. *Int J Radiat Oncol Biol Phys* 2007;68:971–977.

116. Bauman G, Yartsev S, Fisher B, et al. Simultaneous infield boost with helical tomotherapy for patients with 1 to 3 brain metastases. *Am J Clin Oncol* 2007;30: 38–44.

117. Soltys S, Adler J, Lipani J, et al. Stereotactic radiosurgery of the post-operative resection cavity for brain metastases. In: 8th International Stereotactic Radiosurgery Society Congress; 2007 June 23–27; San Francisco, CA. Abstract OS 3-1-1.

118. Yau T, Swanton C, Chua S, et al. Incidence, pattern and timing of brain metastases among patients with advanced breast cancer treated with trastuzumab. *Acta Oncol* 2006;45:196–201.

119. Kirsch DG, Loeffler JS. Brain metastases in patients with breast cancer: New horizons. *Clin Breast Cancer* 2005;6;115–124.

120. Moy B, Goss PE. Lapatinib: Current status and future directions in breast cancer. *The Oncologist* 2006;11:1047–1057.

121. Lin NU, Bellon JR, Winer EP. CNS metastases in breast cancer. *J Clin Oncol* 2004;22: 3608–3617.

122. Lapatinib in combination with radiation therapy in patients with brain metastases from HER2-positive breast cancer. Available at: http://clinicaltrials.gov/ show/NCT00470847. Accessed July 1, 2007.

123. Russell AH, Pajak TE, Selim HM, et al. Prophylactic cranial irradiation for lung cancer patients at high risk for development of cerebral metastasis: Results of a prospective randomized trial conducted by the Radiation Therapy Oncology Group. *Int J Radiat Oncol Biol Phys* 1991;21:637–643.

124. Miller TP, Crowley JJ. Mira J, et al. A randomized trial of chemotherapy and radiotherapy for stage III non-small cell lung cancer. *Cancer Therapeutics* 1998; 4:229–236.

125. Umsawasdi T, Valdivieso M, Chen TT, et al. Role of elective brain irradiation during combined chemoradiotherapy for limited disease non-small cell lung cancer. *J Neurooncol* 1984;2:253–259.

126. Cox JD, Stanley K, Petrovich Z, et al. Cranial irradiation in cancer of the lung of all cell types. *JAMA* 1981;245:469–472.

127. Lester FA, MacBeth FR, Coles B. Prophylactic cranial irradiation for preventing metastases in patients undergoing radical treatment for non-small-cell lung cancer: A Cochrane review. *Int. J Radiat Oncol Biol Phys* 2005;63:690–694.

128. [RTOG] Radiation Therapy Oncology Group. "RTOG Active Protocols." http://rtog.org/members/protocols/0214/0214.pdf. Accessed March 27, 2007.

129. Shu, HK, Sneed PK, Shiau CY, et al. Factors influencing survival after Gamma Knife radiosurgery for patients with single and multiple brain metastases. *Cancer J Sci AM* 1996;2: 335–342.

130. Neider C, Nestle U, Motaref B, et al. Prognostic factors in brain metastases: Should patients be selected for aggressive treatment according to recursive partitioning analysis (RPA) classes? *Int J Radiat Oncol Biol Phys* 2000;46:297–302.

131. Lock M, Chow E, Pond GR, et al. Prognostic factors in brain metastases: Can we determine patients who do not benefit from whole-brain radiotherapy? *Clin Oncol* 2004;16: 332–338.

132. Borgelt B, Gelber R, Larson M, et al. Ultra-rapid high dose irradiation schedules for the palliation for brain metastases: Final results of the first two studies by the Radiation Therapy Oncology Group. *Int J Radiat Oncol Biol Phys* 1981;7: 1633–1638.

133. Kurtz JM, Gelber R, Brady LW, et al. The palliation of brain metastases in a favourable patient population: A randomized clinical trial by the Radiation Therapy Oncology Group. *Int J Radiat Oncol Biol Phys* 1981;7:891–895.

134. Murray KJ, Scott C, Greenberg H, et al. A randomized phase III study of accelerated hyperfractionation versus standard in patients with unresected brain metastases: a report of the Radiation Therapy Oncology Group (RTOG) 9104. *Int J Radiat Oncol Biol Phys* 1997;39:571–574.

# 3

# Prognosis of Patients with Brain Metastases Who Undergo Radiation Therapy

James B. Yu

Jonathan P.S. Knisely

---

The prognosis of patients with brain metastases can be difficult to predict, but long-term survivors are very rare. Five-year survivors are rare (2.5 percent), and ten-year survivors are extremely rare (<1 percent) (1). For this reason, therapy for brain metastases must balance appropriately aggressive therapy with considerations regarding individual patient's wishes and quality of life. To help physicians select the appropriate individualized aggressive therapy for each patient based on the probability of prolonged survival, multiple prognostic indexes have been created and will be discussed in this chapter. In addition, the acute and chronic sequelae from whole brain radiation therapy (WBRT) and from stereotactic radiosurgery (SRS) will be discussed.

## Prognostic Indexes

To help in the prediction of patient survival, several groups of investigators have created prognostic indices. The most frequently used and validated index is the Radiation Therapy Oncology Group (RTOG) recursive partitioning analysis (RPA), which was created from an analysis of the 1,200 patients enrolled in three RTOG trials conducted from 1979 to 1993 (2). Based on this statistical analysis, three RTOG RPA classes were suggested involving four factors: 1) Age <65 or >=65, 2) Karnofsky performance status (KPS) ≥70 or <70 (Table 3.1), 3) Controlled or uncontrolled primary tumor, and 4) Presence or absence of extracranial metastases (Table 3.2). RPA Class I included patients <65 years old, KPS >70, with a controlled primary, and no evidence of

TABLE 3.1 Karnofsky Performance Status

| | |
|---|---|
| 100 | Normal, no signs of disease |
| 90 | Capable of normal activity, few symptoms or signs of disease |
| 80 | Normal activity with some difficulty, some symptoms or signs |
| 70 | Caring for self, not capable of normal activity or work |
| 60 | Requiring some help, can take care of most personal requirements |
| 50 | Requiring help often, requiring frequent medical care |
| 40 | Disabled, requiring special care and help |
| 30 | Severely disabled, hospital admission indicated but no risk of death |
| 20 | Very ill, urgently requiring admission and supportive measures or treatment |
| 10 | Moribund, rapidly progressive fatal disease processes |
| 0 | Death |

extracranial metastases. RPA Class III included patients with KPS≤70. RPA Class II included all the remaining patients. The median survival time associated with the RTOG RPA classes according to the initial (and largest) study were as follows: Class I–7.1 months, Class II–4.3 months, and Class III–2.3 months. This RTOG RPA classification was validated retrospectively (3) and has been extensively investigated in multiple clinical scenarios, with multiple interventions and histologies (Table 3.3). For example, the RPA stratification has been validated with an examination of patients who had been randomized in RTOG 91-04, a trial that examined accelerated hyperfractionation versus accelerated fractionation of radiotherapy for brain metastases (4). For RPA Class I, the 91-04 trial showed a median survival of 6.2 months; for Class II, the median survival was 3.8 months.

The RPA has additionally been validated in patients who have undergone surgery followed by whole-brain radiotherapy (WBRT), with investigators

TABLE 3.2 RTOG Recursive Partitioning Analysis (RPA) Classification

| | CRITERIA |
|---|---|
| RPA Class I | Age <65<br>Extracranial metastases not present<br>Primary tumor controlled<br>KPS >70 |
| RPA Class III | KPS <70 |
| RPA Class II | Not in Class I or Class III |

TABLE 3.3 RTOG RPA for Brain Metastases—Validation Studies

| AUTHOR | N | STUDY FOCUS/ INITIAL TREATMENT | RPA CLASS I MEDIAN SURVIVAL (MONTHS) | RPA CLASS II MEDIAN SURVIVAL (MONTHS) | RPA CLASS III MEDIAN SURVIVAL (MONTHS) | P VALUE |
|---|---|---|---|---|---|---|
| Gaspar et al. 1997 (2) | 1200 | Original RTOG RPA Study | 7.1 | 4.2 | 2.3 | N/A |
| Nieder et al. 2000 (3) | 528 | All patients | 10.5 | 3.5 | 2.0 | <0.05 |
| Gaspar et al. 2000 (4) | 445 | RTOG 9104 patients (Hyperfraction- ation vs. Standard Tx) | 6.2 | 3.8 | N/A | <0.0001 |
| Kocher et al. 2004 (55) | 138 | WBRT | 9 | 4.1 | 2.5 | Not reported |
| Saito et al. 2006 (51) | 270 | WBRT ± surgery | 6.2 | 4.2 | 3.0 | <0.0001 |
| Agboola et al. 1998 (5)[5] | 125 | Surgery + WBRT | 14.8 | 9.9 | 6.0 | 0.0002 |
| Regine et al. 2004 (52) | 95 | Single brain metastases, Surgery ± WBRT | 10.9 | 9.8 | N/A | 0.45 |
| Tendulkar et al. 2006 (53) | 271 | Surgery ± adjuvant therapy | 21.4 | 9.0 | 9.0 | <0.001 |
| Paek et al. 2005 (54) | 208 | Surgery ± adjuvant therapy | 16.1 | 7.2 | 1.4 | <0.002 |
| Sneed et al. 2002 (14) | 268 | SRS | 14 | 8.2 | 5.3 | <0.001* |
| Chidel et al. 2000 (6) | 135 | SRS | 11.2 | 6.9 | 6.9 | 0.016 |
| Lorenzoni et al. 2004 (11) | 110 | SRS ± WBRT | 27.6 | 10.7 | 2.8 | <0.0001 |
| Devriendt et al. 2007 (25) | 267 | SRS | 22 | 12 | 3 | <0.0001 |
| Kocher et al. 2004 (55) | 117 | SRS | 25.4 | 5.9 | 4.2 | Not reported |
| Sneed et al. 2002 (14) | 301 | SRS ± WBRT | 15.2 | 7 | 5.5 | <0.001* |
| Sanghavi et al. 2001(56) | 502 | SRS + WBRT | 16.1 | 10.3 | 8.7 | 0.000007 |

*(continued on next page)*

TABLE 3.3 RTOG RPA for Brain Metastases—Validation Studies (continued)

| AUTHOR | N | STUDY FOCUS/ INITIAL TREATMENT | RPA CLASS I MEDIAN SURVIVAL (MONTHS) | RPA CLASS II MEDIAN SURVIVAL (MONTHS) | RPA CLASS III MEDIAN SURVIVAL (MONTHS) | P VALUE |
|---|---|---|---|---|---|---|
| Weltman et al. 2000 (57) | 65 | SRS ± WBRT | 20.19 | 7.75 | 3.38 | 0.0131 |
| Nam, et al. 2005 (23) | 84 | 1–3 metastases, SRS | 72 weeks | 36 weeks | 19 weeks | Not reported |
| Serizawa et al. 2007 (58) | 752 | 1–4 metastases, SRS | 3.34 years | 1.23 years | 0.74 years | Not reported |
| Viani et al. 2007 (59) | 171 | Breast cancer, WBRT | 11.7 | 6.2 | 3.0 | <0.0001 |
| Muacevic et al. 2004 (60) | 151 | Breast cancer, SRS ± WBRT | 34.9 | 9.1 | 7.9 | <0.0001 |
| Harrison et al. 2003 (61) | 65 | Melanoma | 6.5 | 3.5 | 2.5 | 0.0098 |
| Buchsbaum et al. 2002 (62) | 74 | Melanoma | 10.5 | 5.9 | 1.8 | <0.0001 |
| Radbill et al. 2004 (63) | 51 | Melanoma, SRS ± WBRT | 57 weeks | 20 weeks | 20 weeks | 0.003 |
| Mathieu et al. 2006 (64) | | Melanoma, SRS | 12.7 | 4.9 | 2.3 | <0.0005 |
| Gonzalez-Martinez et al. 2002 (65) | 24 | Melanoma, SRS | 5.9 | 3.7 | 3 | Not reported |
| Chang et al. 2005 (66) | 189 | Melanoma, sarcoma, and renal cell carcinomas, SRS ± WBRT | 9.5 | 7.5 | 2.99 | 0.002 |
| Cannady et al. 2004 (67) | 46 | Renal cell carcinoma | 8.5 | 3 | 9.6 | 0.0834 |
| Muacevic et al. 2004 (68) | 85 | Renal cell carcinoma, SRS | 24.2 | 9.2 | 7.5 | 0.04 ** |
| Rodrigus et al. 2001(69) | 250 | Non-small cell lung cancer | 4.8 | 2.8 | 2 | 0.0029 |
| Galbas et al. 2006 (70) | 72 | Non-small cell lung cancer | 7 | 5 | 3 | Not reported |
| Videtec et al. 2007 (71) | 154 | Small cell lung cancer | 8.6 | 4.2 | 2.3 | 0.0023 |

*(continued on next page)*

TABLE 3.3  RTOG RPA for Brain Metastases—Validation Studies (continued)

| AUTHOR | N | STUDY FOCUS/ INITIAL TREATMENT | RPA CLASS I MEDIAN SURVIVAL (MONTHS) | RPA CLASS II MEDIAN SURVIVAL (MONTHS) | RPA CLASS III MEDIAN SURVIVAL (MONTHS) | P VALUE |
|---|---|---|---|---|---|---|
| Kim et al. 2007 (72) | 13 | Epithelial ovarian carcinoma | 26 | 4 | 4 | 0.007 |
| Ogawa et al. 2002 (73) | 36 | Esophageal carcinoma | 17.1 | 4.7 | 1.8 | 0.006 |
| Nieder et al. 2003 (74) | 113 | ≥4 brain metastases | Too small to calculate | 3.6 | 4.2 | <0.2 |
| Nam et al., 2005 (23) | 46 | ≥4 brain metastases, SRS | Not enough patients | 36 weeks | 13 weeks | Not reported |
| Bhatnagar et al. 2007 (24) | 205 | ≥4 brain metastases, SRS | 18 | 9 | 3 | <0.00001 |
| Bartelt et al. 2003 (75) | 47 | Unknown primary | No patients | 6.3 | 3.2 | 0.01 |

*p value reported for entire cohort, SRS alone and SRS + WBRT (n=569)

**p value reported for RPA Class I versus Class II and III. Class II was not significantly different from Class III.

reporting survival of 14.8 months, 9.9 months, and 6.0 months for RPA Class I, II, and III respectively (p=0.0002) (5). These values compare favorably to the values assigned to patients who do not undergo therapy, indicating improved survival in patients who are selected as able to undergo this aggressive therapy. The RPA has also been validated for patients undergoing stereotactic radiosurgery (SRS) (6).

In spite of the large numbers of studies that report survival and other data by RTOG RPA class, RPA classification scheme has been criticized (7). One reason for the criticism is that RPA classes II and III encompass an inhomogeneous group of patients and that RPA Class III is based solely on KPS, which can be a subjective factor. In addition, there is no generally accepted definition of extracranial disease control, nor any generally accepted definition of controlled primary tumor, and this, when coupled with the inconsistent availability of modern staging studies in retrospective series, may cause even more significant heterogeneity in study populations within the same RPA class. Still, the large number of papers that have reported results stratified by RPA class makes the system useful as a general framework, and if carefully applied, the RPA classification scheme is a reliable framework for selection of patients for study.

TABLE 3.4 Score Index for Radiosurgery in Brain Metastases

|  | 0 | 1 | 2 |
| --- | --- | --- | --- |
| Age (years) | ≥60 | 51–59 | ≤50 |
| KPS | ≤50 | 60–70 | 80–100 |
| Systemic disease status | Progressive disease | Partial remission or stable disease | Complete clinical remission or no evidence of disease |
| Number of brain lesions | ≥3 | 2 | 1 |
| Largest lesion volume | >13 cm$^3$ | 5–13 cm3 | <5 cm$^3$ |

Patients are scored for each factor, and the total score is the patient's SIR score.

(From Weltman E, Salvajoli JV, Brandt RA, et al. Radiosurgery for brain metastases: A score index for predicting prognosis. *Int J Radiat Oncol Biol Phys* 2000;46:1155–1161.)

Other prognostic systems have been developed besides the RTOG RPA classification. The Score Index for Radiosurgery (SIR) was developed by Weltman et al. (8), and several studies report that it more accurately predicts survival and other outcomes in patients who undergo stereotactic radiosurgery for brain metastases (9–11). Under the SIR scheme, patients are assigned scores from 0 to 10, based on 5 factors: age, KPS, status of systemic disease, number of brain metastases, and the volume of the largest intracranial lesion (Table 3.4). SIR scores for patients who have undergone radiosurgery have been reported in several papers (Table 3.5). One of the features differentiating the SIR score from RPA class is the accounting for number of intracranial metastatic lesions. This may be an important distinction, as some authors observed that an increasing number of brain metastases treated with SRS has been associated with poorer survival rates (12–14), while some authors have not noted a difference (15–18). Still, most randomized trials investigating the efficacy of stereotactic radiosurgery have required 4 or less lesions for eligibility (18–22). Notably, other investigators have reported that SRS still improves survival in patients with four or more metastatic lesions (23) and that the total volume of brain metastases, rather than the absolute number of metastases, should be considered when determining the prognosis of patients with brain metastases who undergo SRS (24).

A third simplified Basic Score for Brain Metastases (BSBM), suggested by Lorenzoni et al. (11), appeared to be accurate for estimating survival in patients who had undergone radiosurgery, based on three factors: KPS, control of primary disease, and presence of extracranial metastases (Table 3.6). Based on their retrospective study of 110 patients treated from 1999 to 2003, patients with a BSBM score of 3 had yet to reach median survival (55 percent survival

TABLE 3.5 Score Index for Radiosurgery in Brain Metastases

| AUTHOR | N | STUDY FOCUS | MEDIAN SURVIVAL BY SIR SCORE | | | | | | | | | | | P VALUE |
|---|---|---|---|---|---|---|---|---|---|---|---|---|---|---|
| | | | 0 | 1 | 2 | 3 | 4 | 5 | 6 | 7 | 8 | 9 | 10 | |
| Weltman et al. 2000 (57) | 63 | SRS ± WBRT | | | 2.91 months | | | 7.00 months | | | | 31.98 months | | 0.0001 |
| Gaudy-Marqueste et al. 2006 (76) | 106 | SRS – melanoma No WBRT | | | | | 3.44 months | | | 5.95 months | | 7.11 months | | 0.002 |
| Lorenzoni et al. 2004 (11) | 110 | SRS ± WBRT | | | 2.4 months | | 4.6 months | | 10.8 months | | | 27.7 months | | <0.0001 |
| Devriendt et al. 2007 (25) | 267 | SRS ± WBRT | | | 3 months | | 7 months | | 12 months | | | 23 months | | <0.0001 |
| Selek et al. 2004 (10) | 103 | SRS ± WBRT | | | | 4 months | | | | | 7 months | | | <0.05 |
| Goyal et al. 2005 (9) | 43 | SRS ± WBRT | | | 3 months | | | 8 months | | | | 21 months | | 0.00033 |

From Weltman E, Salvajoli JV, Brandt RA, et al. Radiosurgery for brain metastases: A score index for predicting prognosis. *Int J Radiat Oncol Biol Phys* 2000;46:1155–1161.

TABLE 3.6  Basic Score for Brain Metastases

| | BSBM SCORE | |
| --- | --- | --- |
| | 0 | 1 |
| KPS | 50–70 | 80–100 |
| Control of primary disease | No | Yes |
| Extracranial metastases | Yes | No |

A score of 0 or 1 is assigned for each of three categories: KPS, control of primary disease, and whether or not extracranial metastases are present. The total score is the sum of each category score, and ranges from 0 to 3.

(From Lorenzoni, J, Devriendt D, Massager N, et al. Radiosurgery for treatment of brain metastases: Estimation of patient eligibility using three stratification systems. *Int J Radiat Oncol Biol Phys* 2004;60:218–224.)

at 32 months). Patients with BSBM scores of 2, 1, and 0, had median survival of 13.1, 3.3, and 1.9 months, respectively (p<0.0001). Other investigators have not yet validated this prognostic system. This paper was updated in 2007, and patients with a BSBM score of 3 had a median survival of 23 months (25). At this reanalysis, the authors felt that the BSBM was equivalent to the other prognostic systems (RTOG RPA and SIR scores). The BSBM score was also validated in a prospective cohort of 157 patients, and patients with BSBM scores of 3, 2, 1, 0 points had median survival of 27, 13, 7, and 3.5 months (26).

A fourth, novel prognostic index is the Graded Prognostic Assessment or GPA (27). The GPA was produced by evaluating 1960 patients from the RTOG database. Four factors are considered (Table 3.7): age, KPS, extracranial metastases (none, present), and number of metastases (1, 2–3, >3). The GPA, in comparison to the RTOG RPA, SIR score, and BSBM score, was found to be a better prognostic tool for this large cohort of patients. Median survival time for a GPA of 0–1, 1.5–2.5, 3, and 3.5–4 was 2.6, 3.8, 6.9, and 11 months

TABLE 3.7  Graded Prognostic Assessment (Sperduto Index)

| SCORE | 0 | 0.5 | 1.0 |
| --- | --- | --- | --- |
| Age | >60 | 50–59 | <50 |
| KPS | <70 | 70–80 | 90–100 |
| Number of CNS metastases | >3 | 2–3 | 1 |
| Extracranial metastases | present | | none |

A score of 0, 0.5 or 1 is assigned to each of 4 categories, and the sum of these four categories is the patient's score, ranging from 0 to 4.

(From Sperduto PW, Berkey B, Gaspar LE, et al. A new prognostic index and comparison to three other indices for patients with brain metastases: an analysis of 1,960 patients in the RTOG database. *Int J Radiat Oncol Biol Phys* 2008;70:510-4.)

(p=0.001). Further validating studies are necessary before widespread adoption of this prognostic index.

In addition to the prognostic factors that go into the RTOG RPA, SIR scores, BSBM scores, and GPA (age, KPS, number of lesions, status of extracranial disease, volume of largest lesion, control of primary tumor), there are other patient characteristics that are assumed to affect prognosis. Some research suggests that breast cancer histology promotes better survival rates and a better response to radiotherapy (12,28). RTOG 95-08, which randomized patients to WBRT versus SRS + WBRT for brain metastases, provided evidence of an improved response to the addition of boost radiation with SRS for lung primaries (18,29).

Another factor that may improve survival in patients with brain metastases who undergo whole-brain radiation is the early detection and aggressive treatment of brain metastases. A single-institution study of early detection of brain metastases for resected non-small cell lung cancer using computed tomography (CT) for screening purposes showed a median survival for asymptomatic patients of 25 months and a 5 year survival of 38 percent, although these statistics were skewed by a single patient who was alive at 67 months without disease after surgical resection and chemoradiation for a single 15mm metastasis (30). MRIs have been shown to detect brain metastases at smaller sizes and have a higher preoperative detection rate, though no survival benefit has been proven when MRI is compared to CT (31).

Retrospective predictors for long-term survival (>5 years) after a diagnosis of brain metastases included age (younger than 65), control of the primary at diagnosis, no other systemic disease, RPA Class I, and single brain metastasis at diagnosis. In addition, being selected for treatment with surgery or SRS was also retrospectively predictive for long-term survival (1).

## Sequelae from Radiation Treatment

Radiation treatment for brain metastases can result in both acute and chronic toxicity. The most commonly used metrics for reporting toxicity from radiation are the National Cancer Institute's (NCI) common toxicity criteria (32) and RTOG CNS toxicity grading (Table 3.8).

Acute side effects from WBRT may include scalp irritation and skin peeling, alopecia, nausea/vomiting, loss of appetite, fatigue, and occasional hearing loss, most of which disappear soon after the completion of radiation therapy (18).

TABLE 3.8  CTC Version 2 and RTOG Common Toxicity Grading

*CTC  Cognitive disturbance/learning problems*

| | |
|---|---|
| Grade 1 | Cognitive disability; not interfering with work performance; preservation of intelligence |
| Grade 2 | Cognitive disability; interfering with work performance; decline of 1 standard deviation or loss of developmental milestones |
| Grade 3 | Cognitive disability, resulting in significant impairment of work performance, cognitive decline >2 standard deviations |
| Grade 4 | Inability to work/frank mental retardation |

*CTC  Memory loss*

| | |
|---|---|
| Grade 1 | Memory loss not interfering with function |
| Grade 2 | Memory loss interfering with function, but not interfering with activities of daily living |
| Grade 3 | Memory loss interfering with activities of daily living |
| Grade 4 | Amnesia |

*RTOG CNS Toxicity Grading*

| | |
|---|---|
| Grade 1 | Mild neurologic symptoms; no medication required |
| Grade 2 | Moderate neurologic symptoms; outpatient medication required |
| Grade 3 | Severe neurologic symptoms; outpatient or inpatient medication required |
| Grade 4 | Life-threatening neurologic symptoms (e.g., uncontrolled seizures, paralysis, or coma); includes clinically or radiographically suspected radionecrosis and histologically proven radionecrosis at the time of an operation |
| Grade 5 | Death |

Long-term side effects are the subject of continued study. Previously, whole-brain radiation was thought to be associated in long-term survivors with a high rate of dementia, ataxia, incontinence, and even death. DeAngelis et al., in a frequently cited paper, initially reported a high rate of dementia (11 percent) in long-term survivors of WBRT and attributed this to the radiation (33). However, the fraction sizes used during the era reported were often higher (4 to 8 Gy) than the currently accepted standard (2 to 3 Gy). The possible contribution of chemotherapy or other factors, including systemic disease progression, was not assessed. In patients who had lower fraction sizes, toxicity was more acceptable. This is likely due to the radiobiological effect of high fraction sizes on late responding tissues in the central nervous system (34,35). Dementia has also been seen in patients who undergo standard fraction (2 to 3 Gy) treatment, but to higher cumulative doses than are the currently accepted standard, either because of re-treatment or regional boost (1).

Studies with a quick follow-up have found that neuropsychological function was impaired prior to irradiation, possibly due to the presence of the existing metastases or from chemotherapy administered before (36–38) that there is no difference in neuropsychological function as a result of using different techniques (39–41) or that there are only subtle and nondebilitating sequelae, such as mild impairment of memory function (42).

Neurocognitive sequelae have recently been studied prospectively in a trial comparing WBRT to WBRT and motexafin gadolinium (43). This trial utilized 6 neurocognitive tests to assess the subtle changes that are seen in response to radiotherapy. Indeed, recent analysis of the control arm (WBRT alone) of this trial showed an improved survival and neurocognitive function in patients with radiographic improvement in tumor size (44). Good responders, defined as those with aggregate tumor shrinkage of at least 45 percent by volume, showed improved or stable executive function and coordination. In addition, good responders had a significantly longer median survival than poor responders (300 days versus 240 days, p=0.03). This must be regarded as encouraging, especially in comparison to prior reports that indicated worsened neurocognition and memory loss are sequelae of WBRT.

Other follow-up research has focused on patients undergoing prophylactic cranial irradiation (PCI) as opposed to treatment for existing brain metastases. Gregor et al. followed 9 patients with neurocognitive testing for over 2 years and could detect no overall difference in function between patients with small cell lung cancer who received PCI and those who did not (45).

A European review of 64 long-term survivors after PCI suggested that many patients had measurable neuropsychometric deficits though it appeared that effects on quality of life were minor (46). Whereas 95 percent of patients had an Eastern Cooperative Oncology Group (ECOG) performance status ≤1, only 19 percent performed at the level expected for their age and intellectual ability on all neuropsychometric testing. Fifty-four percent demonstrated impairment on two or more tests, suggesting significant cognitive dysfunction.

Kondziolka et al. reviewed the University of Pittsburgh experience (47) and identified 44 patients who had survived for more than 4 years after stereotactic radiosurgery for brain metastases. The median age was 53, and median KPS was 90. In comparison to shorter-lived patients, longer surviving patients had a higher KPS, fewer brain metastases, and less extracranial disease. Interestingly, overall survival was still prolonged in some patients, even with the presence of multiorgan metastatic disease.

Sequelae from stereotactic radiosurgery for brain metastases have been described retrospectively and in randomized trials. Expected acute and chronic toxicity is acceptable with carefully defined doses (48) that are tailored to the volume of the metastases. Acute toxicity that can occur within 3 months of treatment includes fatigue, hearing or ocular symptoms, nausea/vomiting, headache, lethargy, and seizure. Death that occurs within 3 months of treatment due to radiosurgery is extremely rare. Grade 3 or 4 acute toxicity occurs in 0–8 percent of cases (18,22,29,49). Grade 3, 4 or 5 late toxicity, in the form of radiation necrosis, leukoencephalopathy, late seizures, headache, lethargy, cerebral edema requiring outpatient or inpatient treatment, and other sequelae more than 3 months after treatment, were reported as occurring in 10–20 percent of patients, in the context of a dose escalation trial (48). The incidence of radionecrosis has been reported from <1 percent to as high as 11 percent (18,48,50). In randomized trials investigating SRS, late Grade 3 toxicity occurs in approximately 0–3% of treated patients, and Grade 4 toxicity occurs in 0–3 percent (18,22,48). Grade 5 toxicity is very rare when doses of SRS are chosen using the guidelines for RTOG 90-05 (48).

## Conclusion

In summary, patients with brain metastases have a varied prognosis, which is almost uniformly poor, with rare long-term survivors. RTOG RPA classification is a general framework that has been validated for various treatments including surgery, SRS, and WBRT. The RTOG RPA classification can give general recommendations regarding likely survival. For patients who undergo stereotactic radiosurgery, the SIR or GPA score may be more accurate and may also be helpful in identifying patients who may be long-term survivors. Severity of long-term sequelae from radiotherapy is difficult to predict, given possible preexisting neurocognitive deficits, side effects of chemotherapy, and from tumor burden itself. Patients who respond favorably to radiation may actually have improved cognition compared to their pretreatment baseline. However, the goal of any therapy is palliative, as almost all patients ultimately succumb to their disease.

## References

1. Chao ST, Barnett GH, Liu SW, et al. Five-year survivors of brain metastases: A single-institution report of 32 patients. *Int J Radiat Oncol Biol Phys* 2006;66:801–809.

2. Gaspar L, Scott C, Rotman M, et al. Recursive partitioning analysis (RPA) of prognostic factors in three Radiation Therapy Oncology Group (RTOG) brain metastases trials. *Int J Radiat Oncol Biol Phys* 1997;37:745–751.
3. Nieder C, Nestle U, Motaref B, et al. Prognostic factors in brain metastases: Should patients be selected for aggressive treatment according to recursive partitioning analysis (RPA) classes? *Int J Radiat Oncol Biol Phys* 2000;46:297–302.
4. Gaspar LE, Scott C, Murray K, et al. Validation of the RTOG recursive partitioning analysis (RPA) classification for brain metastases. *Int J Radiat Oncol Biol Phys* 2000;47:1001–1006.
5. Agboola O, Benoit B, Cross P, et al. Prognostic factors derived from recursive partitioning analysis (RPA) of Radiation Therapy Oncology Group (RTOG) brain metastases trials applied to surgically resected and irradiated brain metastatic cases. *Int J Radiat Oncol Biol Phys* 1998;42:155–159.
6. Chidel MA, Suh JH, Reddy CA, et al. Applications of recursive partitioning analysis and evaluation of the use of whole brain radiation among patients treated with stereotactic radiosurgery for newly diagnosed brain metastases. *Int J Radiat Oncol Biol Phys* 2000;47: 993–999.
7. Nieder C. Regarding prognostic factors derived from recursive partitioning analysis (RPA) of Radiation Therapy Oncology Group (RTOG) brain metastases trials applied to surgically resected and irradiated brain metastatic cases: *Int J Radiat Oncol Biol Phys* 1999;43: 1170–1171.
8. Weltman E, Salvajoli JV, Brandt RA, et al. Radiosurgery for brain metastases: A score index for predicting prognosis. *Int J Radiat. Oncol Biol Phys.* 2000;46:1155–1161.
9. Goyal S, Prasad D, Harrell F, et al. Gamma Knife surgery for the treatment of intracranial metastases from breast cancer. *J Neurosurg* 2005;103:218–223.
10. Selek U, Chang EL, Hassenbusch SJ, et al. Stereotactic radiosurgical treatment in 103 patients for 153 cerebral melanoma metastases. *Int J Radiat Oncol Biol Phys* 2004;59: 1097–1106.
11. Lorenzoni, J, Devriendt D, Massager N, et al. Radiosurgery for treatment of brain metastases: Estimation of patient eligibility using three stratification systems. *Int J Radiat Oncol Biol. Phys* 2004;60:218–224.
12. Diluna ML, King JT, Knisely JP, et al. Prognostic factors for survival after stereotactic radiosurgery vary with the number of cerebral metastases. *Cancer* 2007;109:135–145.
13. Lippitz B, Dodoo E, Ulfarsson E, et al. Prognostic criteria for patients with cerebral metastases treated with Gamma Knife radiosurgery. In: 8th International Stereotactic Radiosurgery Society Congress; 2007 June 23–27; San Francisco, CA. Abstract OS 1-1-5.
14. Sneed PK, Suh JH, Goetsch SJ, et al. A multi-institutional review of radiosurgery alone versus radiosurgery with whole brain radiotherapy as the initial management of brain metastases. *Int J Radiat Oncol Biol Phys* 2002;53:519–526.
15. Hsiung CY, Leung SW, Wang CJ, et al. The prognostic factors of lung cancer patients with brain metastases treated with radiotherapy. *J Neuro-Oncol* 1998;36:71–77.
16. Murray KJ, Scott C, Zachariah B, et al. Importance of the mini-mental status examination in the treatment of patients with brain metastases: a report from the radiation therapy oncology group protocol 91-04. *Int J Radiat Oncol Biol Phys* 2000;48:59–64.
17. Sneed PK, Binder DK, Larson DA, et al. Radiosurgery for brain metastases from breast cancer: Lack of influence of WBRT or number of metastases on survival or FFP. In: 8th International Stereotactic Radiosurgery Society Congress; 2007 June 23–27; San Francisco, CA. Abstract PL 3-2.
18. Andrews DW, Scott CB, Sperduto PW, et al. Whole brain radiation therapy with or without stereotactic radiosurgery boost for patients with one to three brain metastases: Phase III results of the RTOG 9508 randomized trial. *Lancet* 2004;363:1665–1672.
19. Mintz AP, Kestle J, Rathbone MP, et al. A randomized trial to assess the efficacy of surgery in addition to radiotherapy in patients with a single brain metastasis. *Cancer* 1996; 78:1470–1476.

20. Noordijk EM, Vecht CJ, Haaxma-Reiche H. The choice of treatment of single brain metastasis should be based on extracranial tumor activity and age. *Int J Radiat Oncol Biol Phys* 1994;29:711–717.

21. Patchell RA, Tibbs PA, Walsh JW, et al. A randomized trial of surgery in the treatment of single metastases. *N Engl J Med* 1990;322:494–500.

22. Aoyama H, Tago M, Nakagawa K, et al. Stereotactic radiosurgery plus whole-brain radiation therapy versus stereotactic radiosurgery alone for treatment of brain metastases. *JAMA* 2006;295:2483–2491.

23. Nam TK, Lee JI, Jung YJ, et al. Gamma Knife surgery for brain metastases in patients harboring four or more lesions: Survival and prognostic factors. *J Neurosurg* 2005;(102 Suppl):147–150.

24. Bhatnagar, AK, Flickinger JC, Kondziolka D, et al. Stereotactic radiosurgery for four or more intracranial metastases. *Int J Radiat Oncol Biol Phys* 2006;64: 898–903.

25. Devriendt D, Lorenzoni J, Massager N, et al. Radiosurgery for brain metastases: A 6 year follow up comparing RPA, SIR, and BSBM patients stratification systems. In: 8th International Stereotactic Radiosurgery Society Congress; 2007 June 23–27; San Francisco, CA. Abstract OS 1-1-4.

26. Devriendt D, Lorenzoni J, Massager N, et al. Comparison between retrospective and prospective use of BSBM system's classification with a 6 year follow up for patients with brain metastases treated by Leksell Gamma Knife radiosurgery. In: 8th International Stereotactic Radiosurgery Society Congress; 2007 June 23–27; San Francisco, CA. Abstract OS 7-1-1.

27. Sperduto PW, Berkey B, Gaspar LE, et al. A new prognostic index and comparison to three other indices for patients with brain metastases: an analysis of 1,960 patients in the RTOG database. *Int J Radiat Oncol Biol Phys* 2008;70:510-4..

28. Petrovich Z, Yu C, Giannotta SL, et al. Survival and pattern of failure in brain metastasis treated with stereotactic Gamma Knife radiosurgery. *J Neurosurg* 2002;97(5 Suppl): 499–506.

29. Kondziolka D, Patel A, Lunsford LD, et al. Stereotactic radiosurgery plus whole brain radiotherapy versus radiotherapy alone for patients with multiple brain metastases. *Int J Radiat Oncol Biol Phys* 1999;45:427–434.

30. Yokoi K, Miyazawa N, Toshimoto A, et al. Brain metastasis in resected lung cancer: Value of intensive follow-up with computed tomography. *Ann Thorac Surg.* 1996;61:546–550.

31. Yokoi K, Kamiya N, Matsuguma H, et al. Detection of brain metastasis in potentially operable non-small cell lung cancer: A comparison of CT and MRI. *Chest* 1999;115:714–719.

32. http://ctep.cancer.gov/forms/CTCAEv3.pdf. Accessed 6/26/2007.

33. DeAngelis LM, Delattre JY, Posner JB. Radiation-induced dementia in patients cured of brain metastases. *Neurology* 1989;39:789–796.

34. DeAngelis LM, Mandell LR, Thaler HT, et al. The role of postoperative radiotherapy after resection of single brain metastases. *Neurosurgery* 1989;24:798–805.

35. Thames HD, Withers HR, Peters LH, et al. Changes in early and late radiation responses with altered dose fractionation: Implications for dose-survival relationships. *Int J Radiat Oncol Biol Phys* 1982;8:219–226.

36. Penitzka S, Steinvorth S, Sehlleier S, Fuss M, Wannenmacher M, Wenz F. Assessment of cognitive function after preventive and therapeutic whole brain irradiation using neuropsychological testing. *Strahlenther Onkol* 2002;178: 252–258.

37. Chang EL, Wefel JS, Maor MH, et al. A pilot study of neurocognitive function in patients with one to three new brain metastases initially treated with stereotactic radiosurgery alone. *Neurosurgery* 2007;60:285–292.

38. Meyers CA, Smith JA, Bezjak A, et al. Neurocognitive function and progression in patients with brain metastases treated with whole-brain radiation and motexafin gadolinium: Results of a randomized phase III trial. *J Clin Oncol* 2004;22: 157–165.

39. Arriagada R, Le Chevalier T, Borie F et al. Prophylactic cranial irradiation for patients with small-cell lung cancer in complete remission. *J Natl Cancer Inst* 1995;87: 183–190.

40. Parageorgiou C, Dardoufas C, Kouloulias V, et al. Psychophysiological evaluation of short-term neurotoxicity after prophylactic brain irradiation in patients with small cell lung cancer: A study of event related potentials. *J Neurooncol* 2000;50:275–285.

41. van Oosterhout AGM, Boon PJ, Houx PJ. Follow-up of cognitive functioning in patients with small cell lung cancer. *Int J Radiat Oncol Biol Phys* 1995; 31:911–914.

42. van de Pol M, Velde GPMT, Wilmink JT, et al. Efficacy and safety of prophylactic cranial irradiation in patients with small cell lung cancer. *J Neurooncol* 1997; 35:153–160.

43. Mehta MP, Rodrigus P, Terhaard CHJ, et al. Survival and neurologic outcomes in a randomized trial of motexafin gadolinium and whole brain radiation therapy in brain metastases. *J Clin Oncol* 2003;21:2529–2536.

44. Jing L, Bentzen SM, Renschler M. Regression After whole-brain radiation therapy for brain metastases correlates with survival and improved neurocognitive function. *J Clin Oncol* 2007; 25:1260–1266.

45. Gregor, A. Cull and R.J. Stephens et al., Prophylactic cranial irradiation is indicated following complete response to induction therapy in small cell-lung cancer: Results of a multicentre randomised trial. United Kingdom Coordinating Committee for Cancer Research (UKCCCR) and the European Organization for Research and Treatment of Cancer (EORTC). *Eur J Cancer* 1997;33:1752–1758.

46. Cull A, Gregor A, Hopwood P, et al. Neurological and cognitive impairment in long-term survivors of small cell lung cancer. *Eur J Cancer* 1994;30A:1067–1074.

47. Kondziolka D, Martin JJ, Flickinger JC, et al. Long-term survivors after Gamma Knife radiosurgery for brain metastases. *Cancer* 2005;104:2784–2791.

48. Shaw E, Scott C, Souhami L, et al. Single dose radiosurgical treatment of recurrent previously irradiated primary brain tumors and brain metastases: Final report of RTOG protocol 90-05. *Int J Radiat Oncol Biol Phys* 2000;47:291–298.

49. Manon R, O'Neill A, Knisely J, et al. Phase II Trial of Radiosurgery for one to three newly diagnosed brain metastases from renal cell carcinoma, melanoma, and sarcoma: An Eastern Cooperative Oncology Group study (E 6397). *J Clin Oncol* 2005;23:8870–8876.

50. Flickinger JC, Kondziolka D, Lunsford LD, et al. A multiinstitutional experience with stereotactic radiosurgery for solitary brain metastases. *Int J Radiat Oncol Biol Phys* 1994;28:797–802.

51. Saito EY, Viani GA, Ferrigno R, et al. Whole brain radiation therapy in management of brain metastasis: Results and prognostic factors. *Radiat Oncol* 2006; 1:20.

52. Regine WF, Rogozinska A, Kryscio RJ, et al. Recursive partitioning analysis classification I and II applicability evaluated in a randomized trial for resected single brain metastases. *Am J Clin Oncol* 2004;27:505–509.

53. Tendulkar RD, Liu SW, Barnett GH, et al. RPA Classification has prognostic significance for surgically resected single brain metastases. *Int J Radiat Oncol Biol Phys* 2006;66:810–817.

54. Paek SH, Audu PB, Sperling MR, et al. Reevaluation of surgery for the treatment of brain metastases: Review of 208 patients with single or multiple brain metastases treated at one institution with modern neurosurgical techniques. *Neurosurgery* 2005;56:1021–1034.

55. Kocher M, Maarouf M, Bendel M, et al. Linac radiosurgery versus whole brain radiotherapy for brain metastases. *Strahlenther Onkol* 2004;180:263–267.

56. Sanghavi SN, Miranpuri SS, Chappell R, et al. Radiosurgery for patients with brain metastases: A multi-institutional analysis, stratified by the RTOG recursive partitioning analysis method. *Int J Radiat Oncol Biol Phys* 2001;51:426–434.

57. Weltman E, Salvajoli JV, Brandt RA, et al. Radiosurgery for brain metastases: A score index for predicting prognosis. *Int J Radiat Oncol Biol Phys* 2000;46:1155–1161.

58. Serizawa T, Higuchi Y, Nagano O, et al. Gamma Knife surgery for 1–4 brain metastases without prophylactic whole brain radiation therapy. In: 8th International Stereotactic Radiosurgery Society Congress; 2007 June 23–27; San Francisco, CA. Abstract OS 1-1-1.

59. Viani GA, Castilho MS, Salvajoli JV, et al. Whole brain radiotherapy for brain metastases from breast cancer: Estimation of survival using two stratification systems. *BMC Cancer* 2007;7:53.

60. Muacevic A, Kreth FW, Tonn JC, et al. Stereotactic radiosurgery for multiple brain metastases from breast carcinoma. *Cancer* 2004;100:1705–1711.
61. Harrison BE, Johnson JL, Clough RW, et al. Selection of patients with melanoma brain metastases for aggressive treatment. *Am J Clin Oncol* 2003;26:354–357.
62. Buchsbaum JC, Suh JH, Lee SY, et al. Survival by Radiation Therapy Oncology Group recursive partitioning analysis class and treatment modality in patients with brain metastases from malignant melanoma: A retrospective study. *Cancer* 2002;94:2265–2272.
63. Radbill AE, Fiveash JF, Falkenberg ET, et al. Initial treatment of melanoma brain metastases using Gamma Knife radiosurgery: An evaluation of efficacy and toxicity. *Cancer* 2004;101:825–833.
64. Mathieu D, Kondziolka D, Cooper PB, et al. Gamma Knife radiosurgery in the management of malignant melanoma brain metastases. *Neurosurgery* 2007;60:471–481.
65. Gonzalez-Martinez J, Hernandez L, Zamorano L, et al. Gamma Knife radiosurgery for intracranial metastatic melanoma: A 6-year experience. *J Neurosurg* 2002;95(5 Suppl): 494–498.
66. Chang EL, Selek U, Hassenbusch SJ, et al. Outcome variation among "radioresistant" brain metastases treated with stereotactic radiosurgery. *Neurosurgery* 2005;56:936–945.
67. Cannady SB, Cavanaugh KA, Lee SY, et al. Results of whole brain radiotherapy and recursive partitioning analysis in patients with brain metastases from renal cell carcinoma: A retrospective study. *Int J Radiat Oncol Biol Phys* 2004;58: 253–258.
68. Muacevic A, Kreth FW, Mack A, et al. Stereotactic radiosurgery without radiation therapy providing high local tumor control of multiple brain metastases from renal cell carcinoma. *Minim Invas Neurosurg* 2004;47:203–208.
69. Rodrigus P, de Brouwer P, Raaymakers E. Brain metastases and non-small cell lung cancer: Prognostic factors and correlation with survival after irradiation. *Lung Cancer* 2001; 32:129–136.
70. Gulbas H, Erkal HS, Serin MT. The use of recursive partitioning analysis grouping in patients with brain metastases from non-small-cell lung cancer. *Jpn J Clin Oncol* 2006;36: 193–196.
71. Videtec GM, Adelstein DJ, Mekhail TM, et al. Validation of the RTOG recursive partitioning analysis (RPA) classification for small-cell lung cancer-only brain metastases. *Int J Radiat Oncol Biol Phys* 2007;67:240–243.
72. Kim TJ, Song S, Kim CK, et al. Prognostic factors associated with brain metastases from epithelial ovarian carcinoma. *Int J Gynecol Cancer* 2007 Apr 18; [Epub ahead of print].
73. Ogawa K, Toita T, Sueyama H, et al. Brain metastases form esophageal carcinoma: Natural history, prognostic factors, and outcome. *Cancer* 2002;94:759–764.
74. Nieder C, Andratschke N, Grosu AL, et al. Recursive partitioning analysis (RPA) class does not predict survival in patients with four or more brain metastases. *Strahlenther Onkol* 2003;179:16–20.
75. Bartelt S, Lutterbach J. Brain metastases in patients with cancer of unknown primary. *J Neurooncol* 2003;64:249–253.
76. Gaudy-Marqueste C, Regis JM, Muracciole X, et al. Gamma-knife radiosurgery in the management of melanoma patients with brain metastases: A series of 106 patients without whole-brain radiotherapy. *Int J Radiat Oncol Biol Phys* 2006; 65:809-816.

# 4

# Surgical Management of Intracranial Metastases

James L. Frazier
Michael Lim
Jon D. Weingart

Cerebral metastases contribute to an immense health problem because a large proportion of patients diagnosed with metastatic brain tumors will die between 3 and 6 months from the time of diagnosis. Metastases of the central nervous system that are untreated lead to increased intracranial pressure (ICP) resulting in progressive neurologic deterioration and death in one to two months (1,2). Approximately 98,000 to 170,000 new cases of brain metastases are diagnosed in the United States annually (3–6). They are ten times more common than primary brain tumors. According to autopsy studies, the incidence of brain metastases in patients with systemic cancer ranges from 24 to 45 percent (4,7,8). Advances in operative techniques have rendered more brain metastases surgically accessible, but a myriad of factors must be taken into account when deciding upon the overall treatment plan for a patient. The following discussion will focus on the role of surgery in the treatment of brain metastases.

## Clinical Presentation

### Symptomatology

The clinical presentation of patients harboring brain metastases will vary and be contingent upon a variety of factors. Ten percent of patients without neurologic symptoms or signs have metastases that are discovered incidentally with head computed tomography (CT) or magnetic resonance imaging (MRI) (9). Approximately 20 percent of patients with brain metastases will present with seizures due to adjacent cerebral cortical injury (9). Persistent headaches and cognitive abnormalities are among other common symptoms. Headache is the presenting symptom in 40 to 50 percent of patients, and more common with multiple metastases and posterior fossa lesions. Approximately 40 percent of patients may present with focal neurological deficits. The intracranial anatomic location and size of metastases determine the extent of neurologic manifestations.

Metastases adjacent to or located within eloquent cortex produce symptoms corresponding to the function dictated by that area of brain. Nearly 80 percent of intracranial metastases are located within the cerebrum (8,10). Lesions near or situated in the precentral gyrus (Brodmann's area 4), or motor cortex, may cause contralateral hemiparesis or hemiplegia. Those metastases located adjacent to the motor cortex usually produce deleterious effects from mass effect because of large size and/or vasogenic edema. Metastases affecting the postcentral gyrus (Brodmann's areas 1, 2, and 3), or sensory cortex, may cause contralateral sensory abnormalities, and those in the occipital cortex may result in a homonymous hemianopsia. Lesions in the dominant hemisphere frontal operculum, Broca's area (Brodmann's area 44), may affect expressive speech, while lesions in Wernicke's area, which includes Brodmann's areas 39 and 40 and may include the posterior third of the superior temporal gyrus, could produce deficits in receptive language.

Furthermore, metastases to the cerebellum, which account for 15 percent of intracranial metastases may cause gait and/or upper extremity ataxia (8,10). Significant mass effect from size and/or edema may result in effacement of the fourth ventricle that could result in obstructive hydrocephalus and increased intracranial pressure. In addition, mass effect upon the brain stem may produce subsequent stupor, coma, and/or death. Cranial nerve dysfunction may result from brain stem metastases, which account for 5 percent of intracranial metastases, depending upon the location (8,10). Patients may present with diplopia, facial weakness, facial sensory abnormalities, and/or vestibular dysfunction.

Significant mass effect from large supratentorial metastases and/or edema usually leads patients to become symptomatic. Patients may have headaches and/or altered mental status, which may resemble a metabolic encephalopathy, from midline shift and increased intracranial pressure. Hydrocephalus may arise from impingement at the foramen of Monro. Hemorrhage into intracerebral metastases, which is more common with renal cell carcinoma, melanoma, thyroid, breast, lung, and choriocarcinoma, results in transient or permanent

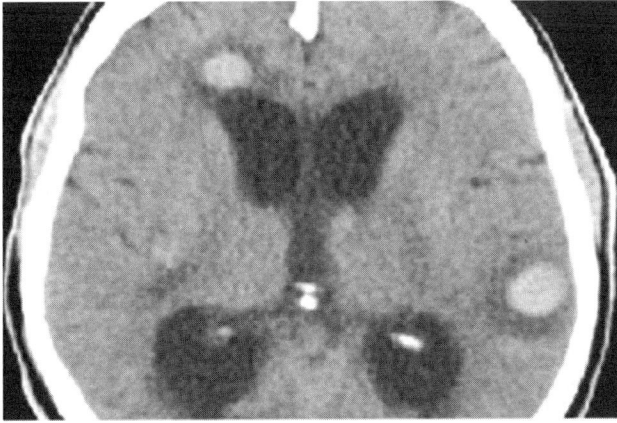

FIGURE 4.1 Noncontrast head CT demonstrating hemorrhagic brain metastases in a patient with known renal cell carcinoma.

neurologic deficits if eloquent cortex is involved (Figure 4.1). In addition, hemorrhage may elicit more edema and a precipitous elevation in intracranial pressure potentially leading to subfalcine and/or transtentorial herniation.

Hemorrhagic cerebellar metastases may also cause significant mass effect upon the fourth ventricle leading to obstructive hydeocephalus from the hematoma and/or the generation of substantial edema. Moreover, a large hematoma and/or significant edema may cause a precipitous decline in mental status from brainstem compression.

## Neuroimaging

The detection and management of brain metastases are usually performed with head CT and MRI. During the CT era (Figure 4.2), approximately 50 percent of brain metastases were presumed to be single, whereas the advent of MRI revealed that multiple metastases can be found in 60 to 75 percent of patients (11,12). A peripheral location, spherical shape, ring enhancement with peritumoral edema, and multiple lesions suggest metastatic disease, but a differential diagnosis should include primary brain tumors, such as malignant gliomas and lymphomas, and nonneoplastic pathologic processes, such as abscess, other infectious processes, tumefactive multiple sclerosis, or stroke. Eleven percent of biopsy specimens of brain tissue revealed primary brain tumors or infections in one prospective study of patients with systemic cancer who were thought to have a single brain metastasis (13).

Acutely symptomatic patients without known brain metastases may present to an emergency department where a noncontrast CT is usually done as an initial diagnostic tool to detect any potential neurosurgical emergencies.

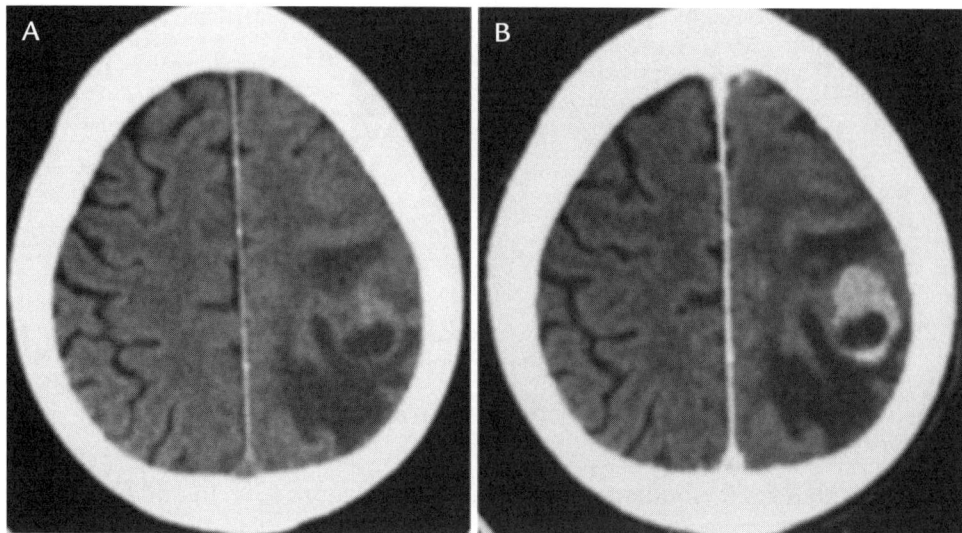

FIGURE 4.2    Noncontrast (A) and contrast-enhanced (B) head CT revealing a brain metastasis with vasogenic edema in a patient with known lung cancer.

Metastases are hypodense or isodense with associated vasogenic edema. Hemorrhagic lesions will be hyperdense. If a brain mass is detected, a contrast-enhanced MRI is the next study of choice. An MRI may be conducted as part of the staging work-up in asymptomatic patients with certain types of primary malignancies, such as non-small cell lung carcinoma.

MRI provides high resolution and excellent anatomic detail of the lesion and adjacent structures. The administration of gadolinium may demonstrate multiple contrast-enhancing lesions situated near the gray-white junction. Without contrast, these lesions may demonstrate mild T1 hypointensity, T2 hyperintensity, and FLAIR hyperintensity. Leptomeningeal metastases are observed as curvilinear or nodular pial enhancement on contrast-enhanced T1W1 and FLAIR images along the basal cisterns or sulci in 35 percent of patients, hydrocephalus in 13 percent, and cranial nerve deposits in 11 percent (14). Patients with intracranial leptomeningeal disease should be further evaluated with imaging of the spine.

Patients with a known primary cancer may present with chronic subdural hematomas that are induced by underlying dural metastases (15). Pulmonary adenocarcinoma, squamous cell carcinoma, systemic breast carcinoma, prostate carcinoma, and renal cell carcinoma can produce dural metastases (Figure 4.3) (16–18).

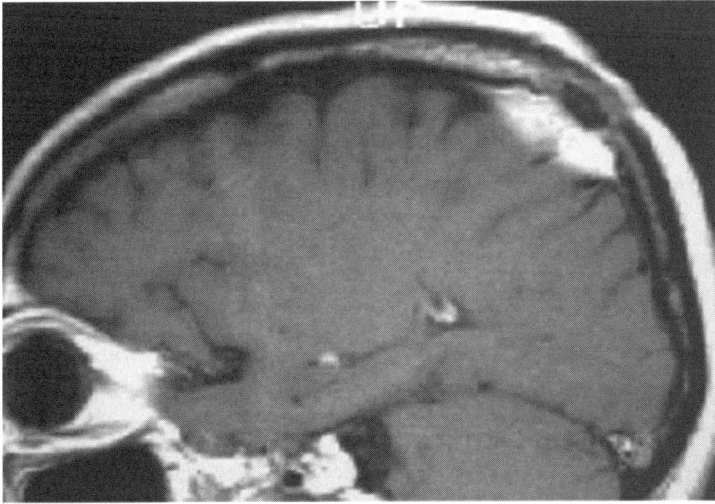

FIGURE 4.3 Sagittal T1 contrast-enhanced MRI demonstrating a dural-based prostate cancer metastasis over the right parietal lobe.

## Patient Stabilization

Headaches and mild neurologic deficits in patients with brain metastases not in extremis are usually caused by edema associated with these lesions. Patients should be started on dexamethasone following an MRI finding consistent with metastases. Dosages vary according to practitioner, but a loading dose of 10 to 20 mg is usually given, followed by 4 to 6 mg every six hours daily. High doses used in the acute period should be tapered to the lowest effective dose as soon as feasibly possible to minimize side effects, such as immunosuppression, hyperglycemia, myopathy, and weight gain. The reduction in symptomatic edema usually becomes clinically evident within 24 to 48 hours after corticosteroid administration. After surgical and/or radiation treatment, the steroids are typically tapered further, although chronic steroid dependence for persistent edema has been observed in patients treated with radiosurgery because peritumoral edema can be exacerbated by radiation effects (19). For those patients with chronic steroid use or extensive edema, a slower taper rate should be used to prevent rebound edema.

Patients presenting with signs of increased intracranial pressure, such as headache, nausea, and vomiting, or alterations in mental status, or with focal neurologic deficits, such as aphasia, hemiparesis, or ataxia, should be evaluated by a neurosurgeon. The findings of mass effect and midline shift, as demonstrated by an initial head CT or MRI, are an indication for immediate neurosurgical evaluation. These patients should be admitted to the hospital and started on high-dose steroids. Patients with acutely deteriorating clinical examinations should be evaluated urgently by a neurosurgeon, since emergent treatment will likely be needed. If the patient's clinical exam acutely deteriorates, intracranial pressure should be managed through intubation, hyperventilation, and the administration of mannitol at a starting dose in the range of 0.5 to 1.0 gm/kg, which can be repeated every four to six hours. Obstructive hydrocephalus, as demonstrated by a head CT, should be managed with the placement of a ventriculostomy for cerebrospinal fluid diversion.

Emergent operative management is usually warranted for large, surgically accessible hemorrhagic metastases, especially those localized in the cerebellum, to reduce intracranial pressure. Deep hemorrhagic metastases, such as those located in the brain stem or basal ganglia, are usually managed medically but should be evaluated by the neurosurgeon.

Patients presenting with a seizure should be placed on an antiepileptic drug to prevent future seizures. For those patients without a history of seizures, the American Academy of Neurology, based upon a meta-analysis, recommends that these drugs should be prescribed only to patients at risk for seizure, and the lowest effective dose should be utilized (20).The data review concluded that prophylactic antiepileptic drugs did not seem to significantly reduce the risk of a first seizure, and side effects were common in 20 to 40 percent of patients. In the immediate postoperative period, antiepileptic medications are given. The length of time varies from a few weeks to a few months.

## Surgical Indications and Patient Selection

### Tumor Histology

Tumor histology plays an important role in preoperative staging because radiation and chemotherapy sensitivities must be taken into account to determine the proper course of initial and/or adjuvant treatment. Staging of the tumor with size, location, and metastases, and grading of the tumor according to histopathologic findings, allow for the estimation of prognosis, and determination of which patients will be candidates for surgical resection. A brain metastasis with a known radiosensitive primary cancer may be suitable for radiation treatment in the appropriate clinical context, such as small size (less than 3 cm) and asymptomatic. Metastatic lesions from small cell lung cancer, germinoma, choriocarcinoma, and lymphoma are very radiosensitive, whereas those from non-small cell lung cancer, breast cancer, and colon cancer are intermediately radiosensitive. Renal cell carcinoma, melanoma, and sarcoma metastases are relatively insensitive to radiation treatment. Metastases from an unknown primary cancer are usually diagnosed by surgical specimens, even after thorough imaging evaluations, and lung cancer is the most common histology.

The most common origin for brain metastases is lung cancer, and approximately 20 percent of patients are affected (21). Up to 10 percent of patients with small cell lung cancer (SCLC) will present with brain metastases, and approximately 50 percent will develop brain metastases during the course of the disease (22). SCLC brain metastases are usually multiple and grow at a rapid rate. Whole-brain radiotherapy (WBRT) is the standard of care for SCLC brain metastases because of its radiosensitivity. Non-small cell cancer (NSCLC) brain metastases typically occur less than one year after diagnosis, and a significant proportion of affected patients have synchronous metastases, in which the metastases present at the time of the lung lesion. The role of prophylactic cerebral irradiation (PCI) has been investigated in patients with locally advanced stage III NSCLC because of the high risk of brain metastasis development, and preliminary results have shown some promise, although more clinical trials are warranted (23,24). A retrospective study analyzed the records of 24 non-small cell lung cancer patients who underwent resection of solitary brain metastases without any evidence of systemic metastases (25). Major prognostic factors were the size of the primary tumor (≤5.0 cm or >5.0 cm), the degree of differentiation of the primary tumor (poor or moderate), operation at the primary site (lobectomy or pneumonectomy), and the elapsed interval between resection of the primary tumor and craniotomy for resection of the brain lesion (≤360 days or >360 days).

In about 5 to 10 percent of patients with renal cell carcinoma, metastases to the brain usually occur two to three years after diagnosis, but may occur several years later (21,26,27). Von Hippel-Lindau syndrome should be considered in renal cell carcinoma patients with a posterior fossa lesion(s) because cerebellar hemangioblastomas are common. Moreover, approximately 7 percent of patients with melanoma develop brain metastases, and they usually occur several years after diagnosis of the primary lesion (21,28,29). As previously mentioned, melanoma brain metastases have a reputation for being radioresistant but have been shown to be sensitive to radiosurgery (30–33).

Breast cancer brain metastases occur in 5 percent of affected patients and are more common in younger patients (21,27,34). They are rarely the only site of metastatic involvement and are typically accompanied by systemic metastases (35). Some brain metastases may be dural-based and mimic meningiomas. Because many systemic metastases are chemosensitive with periodic lengthy survival, aggressive treatment of brain metastases with surgical resection and/or radiosurgery is often advocated (36).

Colorectal carcinoma results in brain metastases in approximately 2 percent of patients, and the posterior fossa is a common location (Figure 4.4) (21,27). These are associated with a poor survival, while brain metastases from esophageal carcinoma are becoming more common due to the improved survival from locally advanced disease (37,38). Both histologic types usually produce cystic lesions that can progress rapidly (35).

Prostate and ovarian carcinomas are rare sources of brain metastases that occur in less than 1 percent of patients. When brain metastases, which have a propensity for the cerebellum and dura, are detected in patients with prostate cancer, these patients usually have systemically advanced disease (39). In contrast, brain metastases from ovarian cancer are often the only metastatic site, and the median time between diagnosis of the primary lesion and metastasis is approximately two years (40,41).

The role of primary tissue histology in determining overall outcome was emphasized in a retrospective study that analyzed 187 consecutive patients

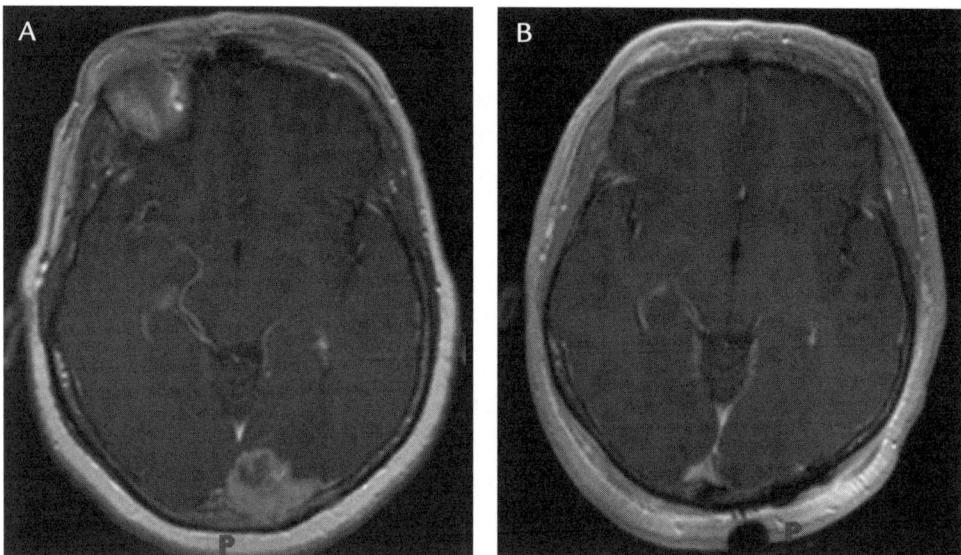

FIGURE 4.4    Preoperative (A) and postoperative (B) T1 contrast-enhanced axial MR images in a patient with a left occipital colorectal carcinoma metastasis.

who underwent surgical resection of brain metastases (42). The primary cancers included lung cancer (85), gastrointestinal cancer (20), renal cell cancer (19), breast cancer (17), malignant melanoma (8), and 38 cases of various other carcinomas, including those of unknown primary site. Of these 187 patients, 111 received WBRT after tumor resection. The presence of systemic disease, preoperative Karnofsky performance status (KPS), lesion number, lesion size, location, nature of adjuvant radiation therapy, and histology of the primary tumor were evaluated as prognostic indicators. Tumor histology had the most significant influence on survival time, and breast cancer patients exhibited the longest survival time, while patients with metastases from renal cell cancer and malignant melanoma had the worst prognosis.

## Lesion Size

When deciding upon a treatment modality for brain metastases, the size of the lesion must be taken into consideration. Operative resection is the preferred treatment modality for tumors larger than 3 cm in maximum diameter. The goal of surgery is to relieve the mass effect, improve neurologic deficits, and achieve local tumor control. Radiosurgery is usually performed for lesions smaller than 1 cm. For lesions between 1 and 3 cm, no prospective randomized studies have demonstrated clinical superiority of either surgical resection or radiosurgery. Radiosurgery should be performed for those patients with a poor KPS score, extensive systemic disease, or for high-risk surgical candidates. Otherwise, surgical resection should be considered for this group, especially if a lesion has extensive peritumoral edema that could be exacerbated with radiation treatment (Figure 4.5) (13).

## Patient Selection

Patients with brain metastases should have a carefully tailored treatment plan because not all patients will benefit from surgical resection of their lesions. Nearly 50 percent of patients with one or two metastases will not be candidates for surgery because of extensive systemic disease, lack of metastasis surgical accessibility, or other factors. Traditionally, patient selection has been based upon who will benefit from surgery and will utilize criteria that includes good performance function as assessed by the Karnofsky performance scale (KPS) score, a single and surgically accessible metastasis, and stable or absent

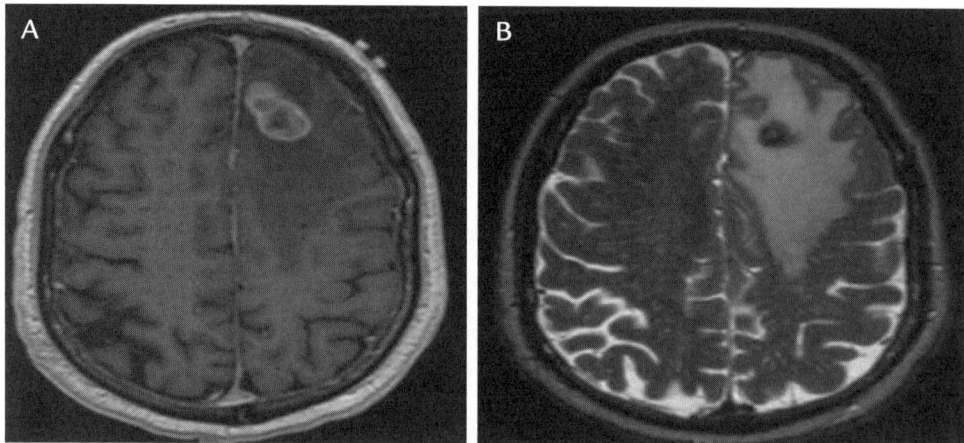

FIGURE 4.5   T1 contrast-enhanced (A) and T2-weighted (B) axial MRI demonstrating a left frontal lobe renal cell cancer metastasis with extensive peritumoral edema. The patient underwent surgical resection of this lesion.

extracranial metastases (43). The KPS ranks patients on their ability to execute activities of daily life, with scores of 70 or above having the best outcome (44). Life expectancy based on systemic disease should be greater than three months for surgery to have a survival benefit. Recently, a new classification scheme has been proposed to categorize patients according to suitability for surgical resection of brain metastases.

The Radiation Therapy Oncology Group (RTOG) developed the recursive partitioning analysis (RPA) class, a statistical method of classifying patients that includes KPS score, patient age, and the status and extent of extracranial disease, based upon the investigation of 1,200 patients with brain metastases (45). RPA Class I patients are characterized by age (65 years or less), a KPS score of 70 or higher, and the absence of extracranial metastases, with good control of systemic disease. These patients are considered the best candidates for surgical resection. Patients in RPA Class II have a KPS score of 70 or higher but may also be older than 65 and have uncontrolled systemic disease and other systemic metastases. Consideration of surgical extirpation of their brain metastases requires analysis of operative risks and duration of survival. RPA Class III patients have a KPS score less than 70, have the poorest prognosis, and are usually regarded as poor surgical candidates (46). The status of the primary disease is usually evaluated with positron emission tomography (PET) and CT scans of the chest, abdomen, and pelvis, in addition to a bone scan and quantitative measurement of serum tumor markers, if applicable (47).

Several other important factors need to be taken into consideration in addition to the RPA classification for the surgical decision-making process. A symptomatic patient may require surgical resection if there is significant mass effect that may be life-threatening, to provide immediate symptom relief and to improve the quality of life. Patients with extensive peritumoral edema and refractory seizures may benefit from resection of the lesion(s). Surgical resection is also warranted in cases in which confirmation of tissue histology is necessary.

The surgical accessibility and location of the lesion are of critical importance when determining the operative candidacy of patients with brain metastases. Unless contraindicated, brain MR imaging is the study of choice for localization of the lesion and assessing its proximity to eloquent cortex. Modern microneurosurgical techniques have minimized the number of regions within the brain considered inaccessible to the surgeon. However, a fine distinction must be made between resectability and accessibility. Factors that determine resectability are whether the tumor is deep or superficial, and whether it is within or near eloquent cortex. Metastases located within or adjacent to eloquent cortex, such as the motor cortex, Broca's area, and Wernicke's area, are generally associated with a higher surgical morbidity than those located in noneloquent cortex (Figure 4.6). Surgical resection of lesions in the thal-

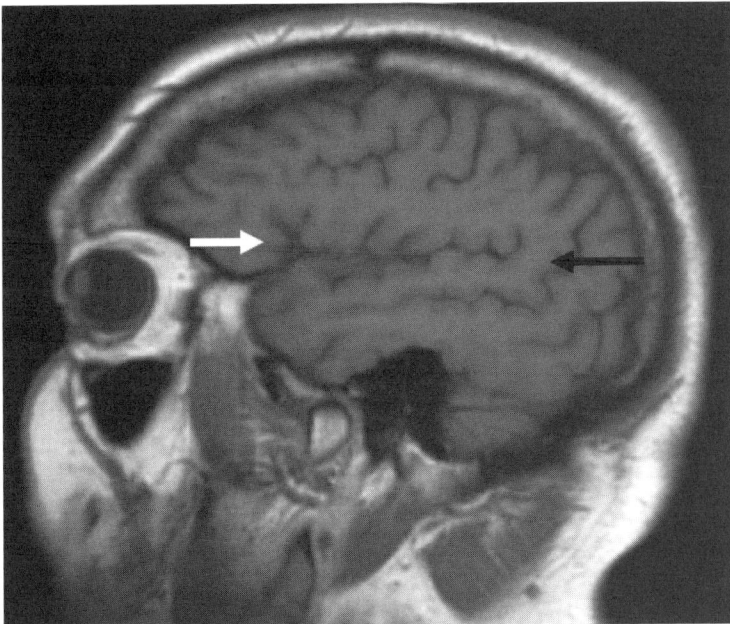

FIGURE 4.6  Sagittal T1 MRI demonstrating general regions of Broca's speech area (white arrow) and Wernicke's receptive speech area (black arrow).

amus, brain stem, and basal ganglia are associated with a higher morbidity and surgical treatment is recommended rarely.

Surgery is contradaindicated in patients harboring leptomeningeal disease. A study in 70 breast cancer patients, who underwent craniotomies for the resection of brain metastases, demonstrated that the absence of leptomeningeal disease was an independent predictor of prolonged survival (36).

## Biopsy

For those brain metastases that are not amenable to surgical extirpation, or for patients with a high operative risk, an excisional or stereotactic biopsy may be performed for tissue diagnosis of the lesion. This includes lesions in the brain stem, thalamus, and basal ganglia. Excisional biopsies are utilized for patients in whom the entire lesion can not be safely debulked through a small craniotomy, but a tissue diagnosis is necessary for the appropriate subsequent treatment. Frameless stereotactic biopsies are performed for deep lesions through the utilization of a three dimensional computerized system. For frame-based stereotactic biopsies, multiplanar stereotactic MR imaging is used to plan the intraparenchymal approach. This approach is useful in patients for whom the risk of general anesthesia is high, because this procedure can be conducted with the administration of a local anesthetic with light intravenous sedation.

## Surgical Management

Prior to the advent of CT imaging, operative resection of brain metastases was uncommon. The resection of brain metastases became a standard treatment option during the 1980s, and the annual number of craniotomies for brain metastases in the United States almost doubled between 1988 and 2000 (35,48). Moreover, the in-hospital mortality of craniotomies for these lesions declined from 4.6 percent to 2.3 percent during this time period due to improved surgical techniques and technological advancements in neuroimaging (48).

Patients with brain metastases should have a thorough preoperative evaluation. Patients with a RPA Class I status are favorable candidates for surgery. The finding of brain metastases in a patient with known cancer raises the immediate question of how to treat. Options include surgery, radiation, or a combination of the two. The goal of treatment is to control the disease in the brain so that this component of the patient's cancer does not affect quality of life. Factors that are important in considering surgery include tumor histology, solitary or multiple lesions, lesion location, and status of systemic disease. MR imaging is the study of choice to detect multiple lesions, plan the craniotomy, and quantify the surgical risk to neurologic function (10,12). Surgical risk must be ascertained through an extensive medical evaluation by performing a thorough history, physical examination, and preanesthesia work-up. In patients with neurologic deficits, the administration of preoperative corticosteroids may assist in distinguishing preoperative deficits related to the tumor in which symptoms may be irreversible from those arising from peritumoral edema that are reversible.

The tumor relationship to eloquent cortex is of utmost importance in assessing the surgical risk. Lesions located in or adjacent to these vital areas of function carry more potential risk. However, tumors can be safely removed even when in eloquent cortex as there is no brain tissue within the metastasis, thus allowing the surgeon to resect safely without harm to the surrounding brain. Therefore, location in or near eloquent cortical areas is not an absolute contraindication to surgery.

A study of 400 consecutive patients who underwent craniotomies for brain tumor resection found that 13 percent of patients had major neurologic complications when the lesion was located in eloquent cortex, in contrast to an incidence of 5 percent and 3 percent, respectively, for lesions located within "near-eloquent" and "noneloquent" cortex (49). Preoperative functional neuroimaging has gained prominence because it assists the surgeon in visualizing the relationship of tumor margins with eloquent cortex and helps determine if the lesion is amenable to surgical resection. Preoperative imaging evaluation begins with MRI with gadolinium. Additional imaging modalities are used to assess the tumor's relationship to eloquent brain areas. Four common imaging modalities utilized are diffusion tensor imaging, functional MRI (fMRI), positron emission tomography (PET), and magnetoencephalography (MEG).

Functional MRI has good spatial resolution and can acquire functional and anatomic images simultaneously. Activation maps reflect hemodynamic variations related to neuronal activity, in which blood oxygen level-dependent imaging assesses changes in local tissue oxygenation to exploit magnetic property changes of hemoglobin as an intrinsic contrast agent. Patients are instructed to perform tasks pertinent to a specific functional area of interest, which should produce a signal on fMRI. A potential complicating factor is artifact related to misregistration caused by patient motion that can be corrected to a certain degree with the analysis software. This modality is advantageous in that it can interrogate the entire brain and be utilized for patients unable to undergo an awake craniotomy for lesions in or near Broca's or Wernicke's areas. Language testing with fMRI has exhibited an 85 to 87 percent correlation of activation areas to within 1 cm of language identified by direct cortical electrical stimulation (DCES) (50,51). Patients can perform receptive speech paradigms by reading and/or confrontation naming for lesions impairing language comprehension located in Wernicke's area. Productive speech paradigms can be performed by patients with lesions impairing speech production, or located in Broca's area. Visual or aural multiple-choice questions are administered for patients with lesions that cause fluent aphasia with impaired comprehension but preserved repetition. The motor cortex, or precentral gyrus, can also be evaluated, but if the patient exhibits motor weakness or impairment, the protocol may be modified with the use of passive or tactile sensory stimulus paradigms in contrast to active sensorimotor paradigms (52).

Functional PET is a nuclear medicine study that can also be utilized to localize eloquent cortex. T1-weighted anatomic MR images are co-registered with PET data, and the contour rendering is performed on the basis of PET data for the eloquent cortex and MRI data for the tumor margins. Magnetoencephalography is a noninvasive technique that measures neuromagnetic signals generated by bioelectric currents within activated neurons. This imaging modality can localize primary sensory cortices and areas involved with receptive language function.

Diffusion tensor imaging (DTI) can assist surgical planning with the identification of intact white matter tracts. This imaging modality constructs maps of the major white matter tracts with tractography demonstrating potential displacement, interruption, or widening of white matter tracts by the tumor. The connections between the eloquent cerebral cortex and subcortical white matter tracts to other areas of the brain and brain stem can be visualized.

## Surgical Techniques

The neurosurgeon endeavors to achieve a gross total resection of the metastasis and obtain clear margins while minimizing the removal of adjacent normal tissue. Most metastatic lesions will have a well-defined margin, which facilitates the microsurgical separation of the tumor from normal brain. Standard neurosurgical techniques employing neuronavigation and microsurgery are used to safely remove these lesions. Patients are usually discharged after 2–3 days.

Tumors in eloquent brain areas can be safely removed if a safe path to the tumor exists. Stereotactic neuronavigation systems are essential, allowing for localization of the tumor prior to skin incision, limiting the size of the incision and craniotomy, and in planning the cortical incision. The surgeon should avoid injury to vessels that may pass through or are located adjacent to the tumor, as they may perfuse normal parenchyma. Subcortical lesions are approached where they are closest to the surface, unless eloquent cortex precludes such an approach. The impact on neurological function of surgical resection was evaluated in a retrospective study conducted between 1989 and 1996 (53). This study demonstrated that the early postoperative KPS score was improved in 59 percent of patients, unchanged in 32 percent, and worsened in 9 percent. In addition, the study's data provided good evidence that function is either preserved or improved with microsurgical resection.

The surgical anatomy must be carefully examined to determine the relationship of the tumor with surrounding structures, as this will dictate the operative approach. Metastases may be categorized according to their relationship to adjacent sulci and gyri (54,55). Cerebellar metastases can be classified as either deep, vermian, or hemispheric, where hemispheric lesions can further be subcategorized into lateral or medial (Figure 4.7). The relationship to adjacent sulci and gyri can be used to classify supratentorial metastases. These lesions

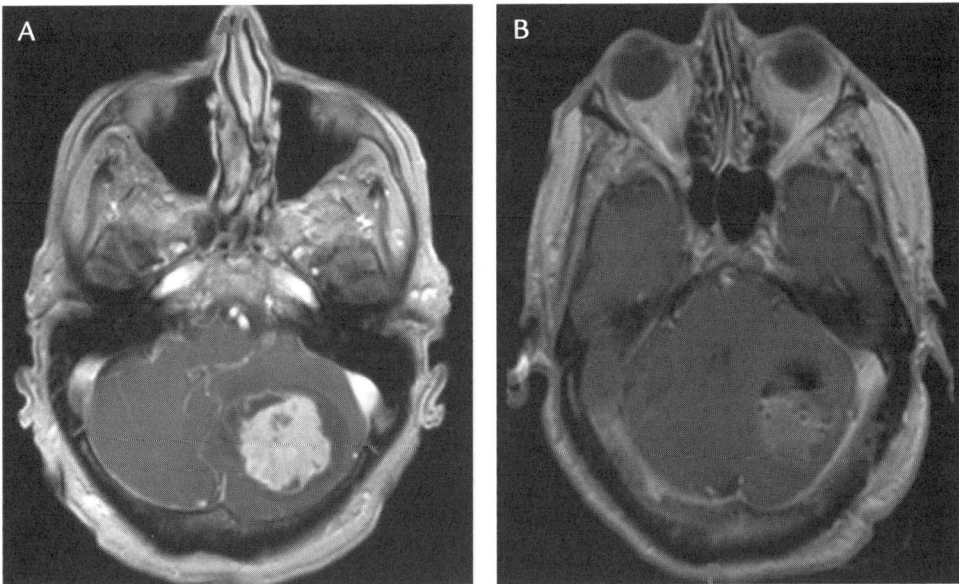

FIGURE 4.7    Preoperative (A) and postoperative (B) T1 contrast-enhanced axial MR images in a patient with a left cerebellar squamous cell carcinoma metastasis.

may be found deep within a gyrus adjacent to a sulcus, under the cortex within a gyrus, deep within the hemispheric white matter, or within the ventricular system.

Patient positioning is vital, because the lesion should be at the top of the operative field. Once the position of the head is determined, it is immobilized in a head-holder, known as the Mayfield 3-pin clamp. The incision and craniotomy can then be planned with a stereotactic neuronavigation system. Moreover, preoperative imaging should be correlated with known anatomic landmarks to localize the lesion to corroborate findings with the neuronavigation system.

Selection of the most optimal surgical approach depends on the location of the lesion and knowledge of the anatomy in the vicinity. For metastases located just beneath the cortex, a transcortical approach with circumferential dissection of the lesion is utilized. Metastases located deep within a gyrus adjacent to a sulcus or deep to a sulcus are typically approached by splitting the sulcus leading to the tumor. The sylvian fissure can be split for metastases located in the subinsular cortex, and the interhemispheric fissure may be split for midline lesions. The transcortical or transsulcal approaches may be utilized for lesions located deep within the white matter. The shortest transparenchymal trajectory is typically used for cerebellar metastases.

Frameless stereotactic neuronavigation is useful in mapping the trajectory to the lesion, in addition to the aforementioned skin incision and craniotomy planning. Frameless stereotaxy is based upon merged preoperative MR images and is fixed in time. Therefore, intraoperative changes, such as brain shift, cannot be accounted for during the operation. Intraoperative ultrasound, which can be used to visualize tumors beneath the surface of the brain, offers the ability of real-time imaging, and changes in the tumor and brain shift can be identified during the operation (56). Solid metastases appear homogenously hyperechogenic, while those with cysts or necrotic centers may be centrally hypoechoic. The value of neuronavigation systems was investigated in a retrospective study which evaluated the postoperative outcome of 49 patients with brain metastases, who had their surgeries conducted with neuronavigational systems (57). Some patients required more than one craniotomy for their lesions. The patients were grouped according to RPA class, and 23 craniotomies were performed for metastases in eloquent areas, while 32 craniotomies were performed in noneloquent cortex. The perioperative mortality rate was 0 percent, and a gross total resection was achieved in 96 percent of patients. For those patients, who were neurologically intact preoperatively, there were no postoperative neurologic deficits. Patients were symptomatic preoperatively in 51 cases, and image-guided tumor resection resulted in complete symptom resolution in 70 percent of patients, improvement in 14 percent, no effect in 12 percent, and neurologic deterioration in 4 percent. With a mean follow-up of one year, the median survival was 16.23 months, and 17.5, 22.9, and 9.8 months for RPA classes I, II, and III, respectively, when further stratified. The local recurrence rate was 16 percent. This study provided evidence that gross total resection of brain metastases can be safely accomplished with a low morbidity rate and improvement of neurologic symptoms with intraoperative neuronavigation systems.

For lesions located in or adjacent to eloquent cortex, intraoperative functional mapping is typically conducted to corroborate the findings of any preoperative functional imaging studies. This will help the neurosurgeon avoid the resection of eloquent brain during the operation and resect as much of the tumor as safely and feasibly possible. DCES, which remains the gold standard, is used to identify eloquent cortex (Figure 4.8). Direct stimulation of the motor cortex elicits a contralateral motor response, which can be detected upon inspection by the anesthesiologist and electrophysiologic signals by a neurophysiologist. Subcortical motor tracts can also be stimulated as the resection of the lesion proceeds deeper near the motor cortex, to help avoid transection of these pathways. During tumor resection, subcortical stimulation of the motor pathways will alert the surgeon that these tracts are in the vicinity, and further resection in the area may result in the loss of a motor response with subsequent stimulation and a

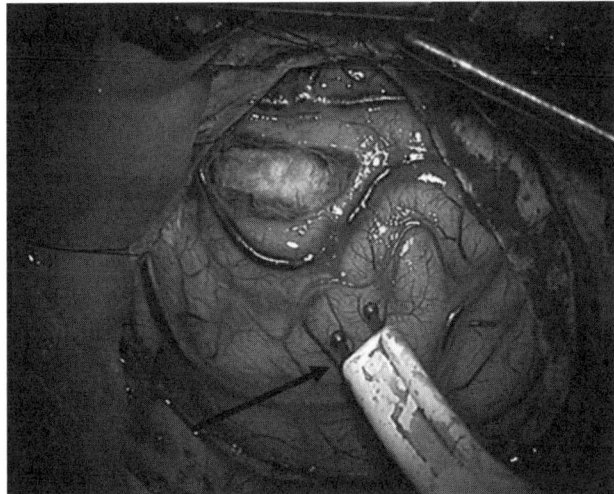

FIGURE 4.8 Use of direct electrocortical stimulation via an Ojemann bipolar stimulator to detect the motor cortex.

postoperative motor deficit. DCES elicits an objective motor response, which has an advantage over using standard neurophysiologic techniques alone.

Somatosensory evoked potentials (SSEPs), a neurophysiologic technique, can provide an indirect localization of motor and sensory cortices. This technique identifies the reversal of phase that occurs between these two cortices. Stimulation of the median, ulnar, or posterior tibial nerves results in cortical potentials that are detected by a strip electrode placed on the cortical surface. A phase reversal is observed when the electrode covers both the motor and sensory cortices because the motor potentials are usually positive and sensory potentials are typically negative. The potentials can be continuously monitored during tumor resection (Figure 4.9).

An awake craniotomy may be performed for lesions in critical language areas. This allows for speech mapping utilizing cortical stimulation to enhance safe resection of the tumor. For intraoperative localization of expressive language, Broca's area, in the frontal operculum of the dominant hemisphere, patients are instructed to conduct sequential number counting while cortical stimulation takes place. Speech arrest occurs when Broca's area is stimulated and number counting is blocked without simultaneous motor responses in the mouth or pharynx. The area(s) can then be marked with a sterile numerical marker for identification during tumor resection. In addition, conversation can be conducted with the patient to ensure that the integrity of this area is main-

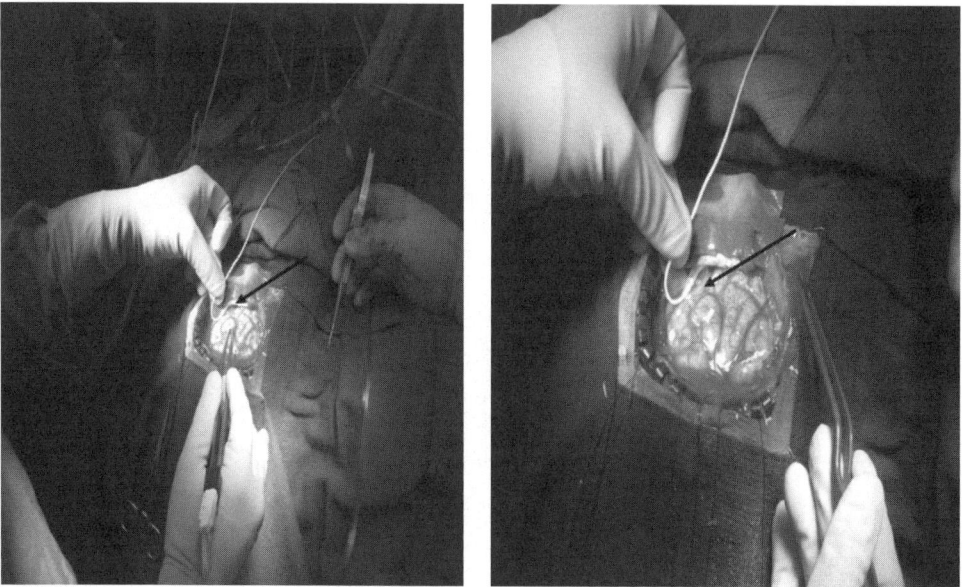

FIGURE 4.9    Placement of a strip electrode for detection of the motor cortex.

tained. Furthermore, receptive language, Wernicke's area, can also be mapped with DCES. During the awake craniotomy, the patient is asked to name a series of objects displayed during cortical stimulation of the area believed to be responsible for receptive language. This area is localized when cortical stimulation prevents the patient from naming an object, and its identity is maintained with a sterile numerical marker, also.

## Single Metastasis

All patients with solitary metastases should be evaluated for surgical resection. The decision for surgery versus radiosurgery is based on the tumor location, surrounding brain edema, and symptoms. Single brain metastases that are large (>3 cm), associated with large peritumoral edema and mass effect, and located in a favorable location should be surgically resected (Figure 4.10). Single metastses causing symptoms or with significant surrounding edema should also be resected. In addition, surgery should be performed in patients with an unknown primary lesion at the time of detection of the intracranial lesion, or the need for tissue diagnosis from a known primary mass. The role of surgery for solitary metastases was delineated in the 1990 Patchell et al. study demonstrating, in a prospective randomized trial, a survival advantage of surgical resection via a craniotomy

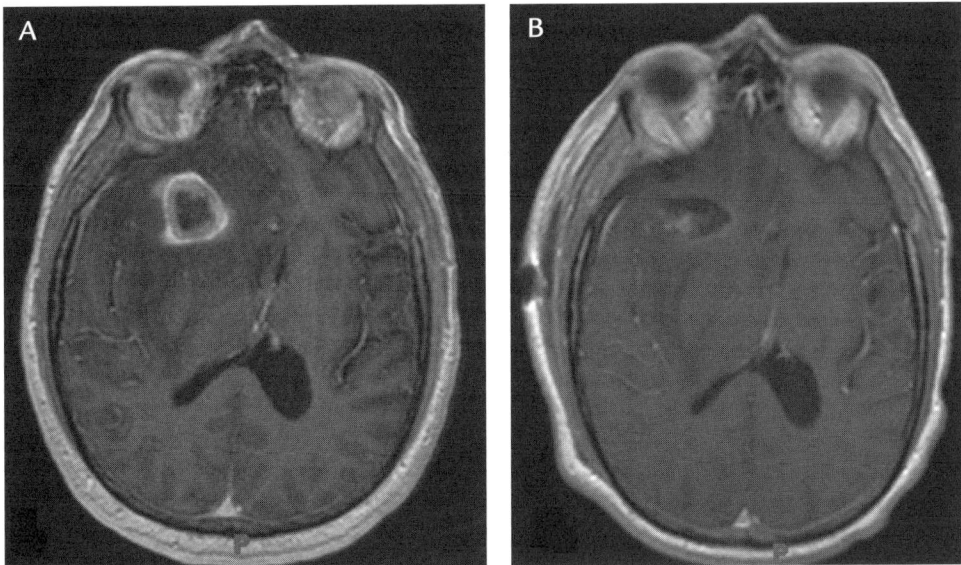

FIGURE 4.10    Preoperative (A) and postoperative (B) T1 contrast-enhanced axial MR images of a patient with an inferior right frontal lobe bladder carcinoma metastasis.

in a comparison of WBRT with and without surgery for patients with a single brain metastasis (13). In this study, which included 48 patients, 25 patients were randomized to a surgical group, defined as surgical resection of the metastasis followed by radiotherapy. The other 23 were randomized to a radiation group, defined as a needle biopsy of the lesion followed by radiotherapy. Patients in the surgical group had a significantly longer survival time (median 40 weeks versus 15 weeks in the radiation group) and longer duration of functional independence (median of 38 weeks versus 8 weeks in the radiation group). Additionally, there was a statistically significant smaller recurrence rate of the metastasis at the original site in the surgical group (5 of 25, or 20 percent) in comparison to the radiation group recurrence rate (12 of 23, or 52 percent). The findings of this study have been confirmed in subsequent analyses. Another retrospective study of 1,300 patients concluded that the treatment modality for brain metastases had a statistically significant effect on survival (58). Patients treated with steroids only had a median survival time of 1.3 months; the median survival time for those treated with radiotherapy alone was 3.6 months and 8.9 months for those treated with operative resection and postoperative radiotherapy.

## Multiple Metastases

Deciding upon surgical candidacy for patients with multiple brain metastases can prove challenging. Metastases with significant mass effect, hemorrhage, or large amounts of brain edema should be strongly considered for operative resection. Patients with four or more brain metastases are usually not treated surgically because the prognosis is typically poor, but a mass effect producing lesion may be removed if there are no surgical contraindications. It is difficult to determine whether aggressive surgical treatment is appropriate in patients with four or more metastases, since RPA class does not predict survival for these patients (59). Surgical treatment should be individualized in this patient population, and the decision to proceed with surgery should be based on quality of life issues. Tumors causing neurologic deficits or elevation of ICP should be considered for resection with a combination of radiation and/or radiosurgery for the remaining tumors.

A recent retrospective study reviewed data on 52 patients with multiple brain metastases treated with radiosurgery, surgical resection, or both (5). The analysis was conducted to ascertain if these patients would benefit from aggressive treatment of intracranial disease. The median KPS score was 90, median age was 58 years, and the median number of brain metastases was 3. Thirty-one patients had radiosurgical treatment alone, 5 had surgical resection, and 16 underwent both treatment modalities. Of these patients, 20 (38 percent) had tumor progression following radiation treatment. The overall median survival was 15.5 months, and RPA Class I patients had a median survival of 19 months. The mean survival for RPA Class II patients was 13 months, and 8 months for RPA Class III patients. Patients with radiosensitive tumors had fewer brain metastatic recurrences in comparison to those with radioresistant tumors. This study concluded that controlled primary disease and a limited number of intracranial metastases in RPA Class I and Class II patients may warrant aggressive treatment.

Another retrospective study reviewed data on 56 patients who underwent surgical resection of multiple brain metastases (60). Group A included 30 patients with one or more brain metastases left unresected, Group B had 26 patients that had all of their brain metastases resected, and Group C included 26 patients with a single metastasis and were selected to match Group B. Group A patients had a median survival of 6 months, while Group B and C patients had a median survival of 14 months. These findings were statistically significant, including the similar outcomes for patients in groups B and C. Similarities were also found in regards to postoperative symptom relief and local tumor recurrence. This study concluded that survival may potentially be improved with the resection of multiple brain metastases.

Operative planning is especially important for the resection of multiple brain metastases. One craniotomy that encompasses all of the metastases may be performed if they are in close proximity to each other, or multiple craniotomies for lesions that are not located in the same vicinity (Figure 4.11). In some cases, the patient may not need to be redraped for multiple craniotomies if the head just needs to be turned from side to side on the operating table.

## Recurrent Metastases

Recurrent metastases should be divided into two groups: 1.) local recurrence, and 2.) distant recurrences. Prognostic factors, such as KPS score and extent of systemic disease are taken into account when evaluating and treating patients with recurring metastases. Local recurrence at a single site in the absence of other brain lesions should be treated aggressively. In patients who received radiosurgery as the primary treatment or as an adjuvant treatment after surgery, an accurate diagnosis based solely upon MR imaging can be difficult. In

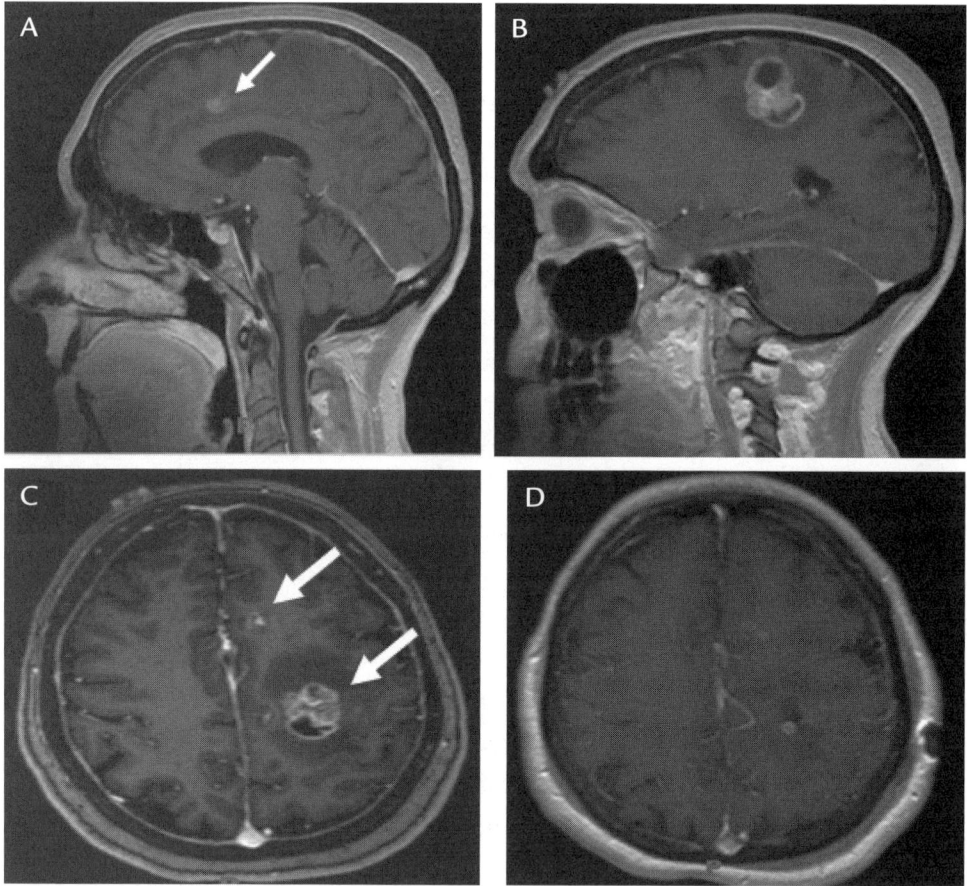

FIGURE 4.11 Preoperative T1 contrast-enhanced sagittal (A,B), axial (C), and postoperative T1 contrast-enhanced axial (D) MR images in a patient who underwent resection of two cervical carcinoma metastases through one large craniotomy.

these patients, tumor recurrence and radiation necrosis can appear similar on an MRI. PET scanning and MRI spectroscopy can be useful in trying to differentiate the two. When there is uncertainty, surgical resection is indicated to remove the enhancing area and establish the diagnosis. The reflex response of giving additional radiosurgery should be avoided.

In patients with recurrences in the brain distant from the original brain site, the overall prognosis is critical in making a decision regarding surgical treatment. Quality of life concerns take priority. If the distant recurrence is solitary, then surgical resection is an option. If there are multiple distant recurrences, then surgery should be offered only for large tumors causing symptoms, mass effect, or with significant surrounding brain edema.

Successful retreatment with surgery in select patients has been demonstrated in some studies. Median survival for patients with recurrence treated with resection was 5 months for 109 patients with NSCLC, 11.5 months for 48 patients with mixed histologies, and 9 months for 21 patients with other mixed histologies in another study (61–63). Patchell et al. conducted a prospective study on 46 patients with a single brain metastasis, who were randomized to receive or not receive postoperative radiation treatment (64). The local recurrence rate was 46 percent in patients without postoperative radiation treatment, and the distal recurrence rate was 37 percent. Local recurrence rates of 10 percent to 15 percent have been found in other studies (65).

## Leptomeningeal Metastases

Meningeal carcinomatosis is being diagnosed more frequently as patients are living longer and occurs in approximately 5 percent of patients. As mentioned previously, the presence of this disease is typically a contraindication for resection of intraparenchymal metastases. The leptomeninges is affected by direct extension from preexisting parenchymal tumor or hematogenous spread of tumor cells, which can then be disseminated throughout the neuroaxis by cerebrospinal fluid (CSF) flow. Metastases from breast, lung, and melanoma cancers are most commonly associated with leptomeningeal disease. Patients usually present with headaches from increased intracranial pressure due to the obstruction of CSF outflow pathways and subsequent hydrocephalus, encephalopathy, seizures or focal neurologic deficits due to direct invasion into parenchyma, cranial nerve palsies, and/or stroke-like symptoms from local ischemia as a result of perivascular infiltration of tumor cells. Analysis of CSF and/or MRI is typically conducted to make the diagnosis of leptomeningeal disease. CSF analysis may reveal pleocytosis, elevated protein concentration, and decreased glucose concentration.

An Ommaya reservoir can be placed in the lateral ventricle via stereotactic neuronavigational imaging guidance for intrathecal therapy. The combination of radiation treatment and intrathecal therapy may increase the median survival by 3 to 6 months in patients with minimal systemic disease and good KPS score (66). The median survival is 4 to 6 weeks without treatment, and death is the result of progressive neurologic deterioration.

# Postoperative Care and Potential Complications

The immediate postoperative period is critical in the care of patients for the detection and/or minimization of potential complications. For patients who are stable in the immediate postoperative period, a contrast-enhanced brain MRI is usually obtained within 24 to 48 hours to confirm gross total resection of the tumor. The extent of vasogenic edema can also be evaluated. For patients with new-onset postoperative neurological deficits and/or decreased mental status, a head CT should be obtained immediately to exclude the possibility of a post-operative hematoma at the surgical resection cavity, subdural hematoma, epidural hematoma, and/or increased vasogenic edema that may necessitate taking the patient back to the operating room for surgical evacuation of the hematoma. Additionally, in the presence of a negative head CT, seizures and/or metabolic abnormalities must be considered.

Seizures occur in up to 20 percent of patients with brain metastases. Many neurosurgeons will utilize perioperative and postoperative prophylactic anticonvulsants for patients undergoing a craniotomy. Patients who are seizure-free preoperatively and who remain without seizures postoperatively are typically taken off of the anticonvulsant(s) with the time course determined by surgeon preference. The American Academy of Neurology has found that administration of anticonvulsants does not provide significant benefit to justify their use on a prophylactic basis in the absence of a history of seizures (20).

The presence of postoperative edema is addressed with corticosteroids that are typically started preoperatively and continued in the postoperative period. Although corticosteroids are advantageous in the acute setting, they have numerous undesired side effects, such as poor wound healing, hyperglycemia, immune compromise, skin changes, fat redistribution, and myopathy. Therefore, depending on the patient's clinical course, the lowest effective dose of corticosteroids should be used and tapered as early as can be tolerated postoperatively.

Venous thromboembolic disease can contribute significantly to surgical morbidity and mortality, and occurs in approximately 15 percent of patients. Patients with brain metastases may be more susceptible to venous thromboembolic disease (67). Low-dose heparin, lower extremity compression stockings, and pneumatic compression boots have been shown to be effective in preventing the development of thrombotic complications. A prospective study provided evidence that mini-dose heparin or unfractionated heparinized components may be safely initiated 24 hours after craniotomy without significant increases in bleeding complications (68).

Surgical mortality has dramatically decreased due to improvements in microneurosurgical techniques. Harvey Cushing found that the mortality after resection of brain metastases was high at around 38 percent in the early twentieth century (69). Surgical mortalities of 3 percent or less were frequently reported in the 1990s, while more recent series have reported a 0 percent mortality rate (56,62,70,71). A retrospective study of 194 craniotomies for brain metastases at a single institution showed a mortality rate of 2 percent, with 2 patients succumbing to sepsis and another 2 patients dying as a result of leptomeningeal disease (49).

Surgical morbidity rates have been reported in the range of 5 to 23 percent, with causes including neurologic problems/deficits, wound infection, postoperative hematoma, pneumonia, deep venous thrombosis, and pulmonary embolism (13,29,60,72–74). The previously mentioned retrospective study, which analyzed surgical mortality in 194 craniotomies for brain metastases, also evaluated postoperative complications in the same group of patients (49). Postoperative complications were classified as neurologic (producing neurologic deficits), regional (surgical site problem), or systemic (general medical issues). Complications were considered minor if they were not life-threatening and were resolved within 30 days without surgical intervention; complications were considered major if they were life-threatening, necessitated surgical treatment, and/or persisted for more than 30 days. Neurologic, regional, and systemic complications rates were 6 percent, 3 percent, and 6 percent, respectively. The relationship of the lesion to eloquent cortex was the most significant factor affecting the rate of neurologic postoperative complications. Patients with tumors in noneloquent regions had fewer neurologic complications than those patients with lesions located within or near eloquent areas. The neurologic postoperative complication rate was found to be 13 percent for patients with lesions located within eloquent brain. Moreover, the study found a 5 percent risk of major complications for patients with a KPS score of 100, a young age range (near 40), and a metastasis not located within eloquent brain. In contrast, a 23 percent risk of major complications was found in patients older than 65, with a low KPS score of 50, and a lesion located within eloquent brain.

## Conclusion

Advances in the operative management of brain metastases have significantly improved treatment options for many patients. Improvements in microneurosurgical techniques, neuroimaging technology, intraoperative computer-guided stereotactic neuronavigation systems, and patient selection processes have been correlated with a better outcome. All patients with solitary metastases should be evaluated for surgical resection. Treatment should be individualized on the basis of prognostic factors, and patients with acute neurologic deficits and/or in extremis require immediate neurosurgical consultation. Tumor histology, staging, grading, and size are important factors, along with KPS score, RPA class, and medical comorbidities, when determining whether or not a patient is a good surgical candidate. Surgical accessibility of the lesion(s) is a critical factor, because a significant number of tumors are not accessible even with the most optimal surgical procedures. The number of brain metastases is currently not an absolute indicator for or against surgery, although patients with four or more brain tumors are usually not treated surgically because of a poor prognosis. Radiosurgery and WBRT are adjuvant treatment options for patients treated surgically for brain metastases.

# References

1. DiStefano A, Yap YY, Hortobagyi G, et al. The natural history of breast cancer patients with brain metastases. *Cancer* 1979;44:1913–1918.
2. Landis S, Murray T, Bolden S. Cancer statistics. CA Cancer J Clin 1999;49:8–31.
3. Larson D, Rubenstein J, McDermott M. Treatment of metastatic cancer. In: *Cancer Principles and Practice of Oncology*. DeVita V, Hellman S, Rosenberg S (Eds). Philadelphia: Lippincott Williams & Wilkins, 2004. pp. 2323–2398.
4. Nussbaum E, Djalilian H, Cho K, et al. Brain metastases: Histology, multiplicity, surgery, and survival. *Cancer* 1996;78:1781–1788.
5. Pollock B, Brown P, Foote R, et al. Properly selected patients with multiple brain metastases may benefit from aggressive treatment of their intracranial disease. *J Neurooncol* 2003;61:73–80.
6. Posner J. Management of brain metastases. *Rev Neurol* 1992;148:477–487.
7. Coia L. The role of radiation therapy in the treatment of brain metastases. *Int J Radiat Oncol Biol Phys* 1992;23:229–238.
8. Posner J, Chernik N. Intracranial metastases from systemic cancer. *Adv Neurol* 1978;19:579–592.
9. Nguyen T, DeAngelis L. Treatment of brain metastases. *J Support Oncol* 2004;2:405–410.
10. Delattre J, Krol G, Thaler H, et al. Distribution of brain metastases. *Arch Neurol* 1988;45:741–744.
11. Schellinger P, Meinck H, Thron A. Diagnostic accuracy of MRI compared to CT in patients with brain metastases. *J Neurooncol* 1999;44:275–281.
12. Sze G, Milano E, Johnson C, et al. Detection of brain metastases: comparison of contrast-enhanced MR with unenhanced MR and enhanced CT. *AJNR* 1990;11:785–791.
13. Patchell RA, Tibbs PA, Walsh JW. A randomized trial of surgery in the treatment of single metastases to the brain. *N Engl J Med* 1990;322:494–500.
14. Collie D, Brush J, Lammie G, et al. Imaging features of leptomeningeal metastases. *Clin Radiol* 1999;54:765–771.
15. Tseng S, Liao C, Lin S, et al. Dural Metastasis in patients with malignant neoplasm and chronic subdural hematoma. *Acta Neurol Scand* 2003;108:43–46.

16. Kleinschmidt-DeMasters B. Dural metastases: A retrospective surgical and autopsy series. *Arch Pathol Lab Med* 2001;125:880–887.

17. Richiello A, Sparano L, Caro MDBD, et al. Dural metastasis mimicking falx meningioma: Case report. *J Neurosurg Sci* 2003;47:167–171.

18. Rumana C, Hess K, Shi W, et al. Metastatic brain tumors with dural extension. *J Neurosurg* 1998; 89:552–558.

19. Boyd T, Mehta M. Stereotactic radiosurgery for brain metastases. *Oncology (Hunting)* 1999;13:1397–1409.

20. Glantz M, Cole B, Forsyth P, et al. Practice parameter: Anticonvulsant prophylaxis in patients with newly diagnosed brain tumors. Report of the Quality Standards Subcommittee of the American Academy of Neurology. *Neurology* 2000;54:1886–1893.

21. Barnholtz-Sloan J, Sloan A, Davis F, et al. Incidence proportions of brain metastases in patients diagnosed (1973–2001) in the Metropolitan Detroit Cancer Surveillance System. *J Clin Oncol* 2004;22:2865–2872.

22. Quan AL, Videtic GM, Suh JH. Brain metastases in small cell lung cancer. *Oncology (Williston Park)* 2004;18:961–972, discussion 974, 979-980, 987.

23. Pottgen C, Eberhardt W, Stuschke M. Prophylactic cranial irradiation in lung cancer. *Curr Treat Options Oncol* 2004;5:43–50.

24. Stuschke M, Eberhardt W, Pottgen C, et al. Prophylactic cranial irradiation in locally advanced non-small-cell lung cancer after multimodality treatment: long-term. *J Clin Oncol* 1999;17:2700–2709.

25. Saitoh Y, Fujisawa T, Shiba M, et al. Prognostic factors in surgical treatment of solitary brain metastasis after resection of non-small-cell lung cancer. *Lung Cancer* 1999;24:99–106.

26. Cimatti M, Salvati M, Caroli E, et al. Extremely delayed cerebral metastasis from renal carcinoma: Report of four cases and critical analysis of the literature. *Tumori* 2004;90:342–344.

27. Schouten L, Rutten J, Huveneers H, et al. Incidence of brain metastases in a cohort of patients with carcinoma of the breast, colon, kidney, and lung and melanoma. *Cancer* 2002;94:2698–2705.

28. Fife K, Colman M, Stevens G, et al. Determinants of outcome in melanoma patients with cerebral metastases. *J Clin Oncol* 2004;22:1293–1300.

29. Sampson J, JH C, Friedman A, et al. Demographics, prognosis, and therapy in 702 patients with brain metastases from malignant melanoma. *J Neurosurg* 1998;88:11–20.

30. Brown PD, Brown CA, Pollock BE, et al. Stereotactic radiosurgery for patients with "radioresistant" brain metastases. *Neurosurgery* 2002;51:656–665, discussion 665-657.

31. Mori Y, Kondziolka D, Flickinger J, et al. Stereotactic radiosurgery for cerebral metastatic melanoma: Factors affecting local disease control and survival. *Int J Radiat Oncol Biol Phys* 1998;42:581–589.

32. Seung SK, Shu HK, McDermott MW, et al. Stereotactic radiosurgery for malignant melanoma to the brain. *Surg Clin North Am* 1996;76:1399–1411.

33. Seung SK, Sneed PK, McDermott MW, et al. Gamma knife radiosurgery for malignant melanoma brain metastases. *Cancer J Sci Am* 1998;4:103–109

34. Chang EL, Lo S. Diagnosis and management of central nervous system metastases from breast cancer. *Oncologist* 2003;8:398–410.

35. Barker FG. Surgical and radiosurgical management of brain metastases. *Surg Clin North Am* 2005;85:329–345.

36. Wronski M, Arbit E, McCormick B: Surgical treatment of 70 patients with brain metastases from breast carcinoma. *Cancer* 1997;80:1746–1754.

37. Weinberg JS, Suki D, Hanbali F, et al. Metastasis of esophageal carcinoma to the brain. *Cancer* 2003;98:1925–1933.

38. Wronski M, Arbit E. Resection of brain metastases from colorectal carcinoma in 73 patients. *Cancer* 1999;85:1677–1685.

39. Tremont-Lukats IW, Bobustuc G, Lagos GK, et al. Brain metastasis from prostate carcinoma: The M.D. Anderson Cancer Center experience. *Cancer* 2003;98:363–368.

40. Cohen ZR, Suki D, Weinberg JS, et al. Brain metastases in patients with ovarian carcinoma: Prognostic factors and outcome. *J Neurooncol* 2004;66:313–325.

41. Tangjitgamol S, Levenback CF, Beller U, et al. Role of surgical resection for lung, liver, and central nervous system metastases in patients with gynecological cancer: a literature review. *Int J Gynecol Cancer* 2004;14:399–422.

42. Kamby C, Soerensen PS. Characteristics of patients with short and long survivals after detection of intracranial metastases from breast cancer. *J Neurooncol* 1986;6:37–45.

43. Sills AK. Current treatment approaches to surgery for brain metastases. *Neurosurgery* 2005;57:S4-24-S24-32.

44. Schag CC, Heinrich RL, Ganz PA. Karnofsky performance status revisited: Reliability, validity, and guidelines. *J Clin Oncol* 1984;2:187–193.

45. Gaspar L, Scott C, Rotman M, et al. Recursive partitioning analysis (RPA) of prognostic factors in three Radiation Therapy Oncology Group (RTOG) brain metastases trials. *Int J Radiat Oncol Biol Phys* 1997;37:745–751.

46. Agboola O, Benoit B, Cross P, et al. Prognostic factors derived from recursive partitioning analysis (RPA) of Radiation Therapy Oncology Group (RTOG) brain metastases trials applied to surgically resected and irradiated brain metastatic cases. *Int J Radiat Oncol Biol Phys* 1998;42:155–159.

47. Lang FF, Sawaya R. Surgical management of cerebral metastases. *Neurosurg Clin N Am* 1996;7:459–484.

48. Barker FG. Craniotomy for the resection of metastatic brain tumors in the US, 1988–2000. *Cancer* 2004;100:999–1007.

49. Sawaya R, Hammoud M, Schoppa D, et al. Neurosurgical outcomes in a modern series of 400 craniotomies for treatment of parenchymal tumors. *Neurosurgery* 1998;42:1044–1055, discussion 1055–1046.

50. Brannen JH, Badie B, Moritz CH, et al. Reliability of functional MR imaging with word-generation tasks for mapping Broca's area. *AJNR* 2001;22:1711–1718.

51. FitzGerald DB, Cosgrove GR, Ronner S, et al. Location of language in the cortex: A comparison between functional MR imaging and electrocortical stimulation. *AJNR* 1997;18: 1529–1539.

52. Lee CC, Jack CR, Riederer SJ. Active versus passive activation tasks. *AJNR* 1998;19:847–852.

53. Korinth MC, Delonge C, Hutter BO, et al. Prognostic factors for patients with microsurgically resected brain metastases. *Onkologie* 2002;25:420–425.

54. Kelly PJ, Kall BA, Goerss SJ. Results of computed tomography-based computer-assisted stereotactic resection of metastatic intracranial tumors. *Neurosurgery* 1988;22:7–17.

55. Yasargil MG (Ed.). *Topographic anatomy for microsurgical approaches to intrinsic brain tumors.* New York: Thieme Medical Publishing, 1994. Vol. IVA.

56. Hammoud M, Ligon BL, elSouki R, et al. Use of intraoperative ultrasound for localizing tumors and determining the extent of resection: A comparative study with magnetic resonance imaging. *J Neurosurg* 1996;84:737–741.

57. Tan TC, Mc LBP. Image-guided craniotomy for cerebral metastases: Techniques and outcomes. *Neurosurgery* 2003;53:82–89, discussion 89–90.

58. Lagerwaard FJ, Levendag PC, Nowak PJ, et al. Identification of prognostic factors in patients with brain metastases: A review of 1292 patients. *Int J Radiat Oncol Biol Phys* 1999;43:795–803.

59. Nieder C, Andratschke N, Grosu A, et al. Recursive partitioning analysis (RPA) class does not predict survival in patients with four or more brain metastases. *Strahlenther Onkol* 2003;179:16–20.

60. Bindal RK, Sawaya R, Leavens ME, et al. Surgical treatment of multiple brain metastases. *J Neurosurg* 1993;79:210–216.

61. Arbit E, Wronski M, Burt M, et al. The treatment of patients with recurrent brain metastases: A retrospective analysis of 109 patients with non-small cell ling cancer. *Cancer* 1995;76:765–773.

62. Bindal RK, Sawaya R, Leavens ME, et al. Reoperation for recurrent metastatic brain tumors. *J Neurosurg* 1995;83:600–604.
63. Sundaresan N, Sachdev VP, DiGiacinto GV, et al. Reoperation for brain metastases. *J Clin Oncol* 1988;6:1625–1629.
64. Patchell RA, Tibbs PA, Regine WF, et al. Postoperative radiotherapy in the treatment of single metastases to the brain: A randomized trial. *JAMA* 1998;280:1485–1489.
65. Sawaya R. Surgical treatment of brain metastases. *Clin Neurosurg* 1999;45:41–47.
66. Buckner JC, Brown PD, O'Neill BP, et al. Central Nervous System Tumors. *Mayo Clin Proc* 2007;82:1271–1286.
67. Schiff D, DeAngelis LM. Therapy of venous thromboembolism in patients with brain metastases. *Cancer* 1994;73:493–498.
68. Kosir MA, Schmittinger L, Barno-Winarski L, et al. Prospective double-arm study of fibrinolysis in surgical patients. *J Surg Res* 1998;74:96–101.
69. Cushing H. Notes upon a series of 2000 verified cases with surgical-mortality percentages pertaining thereto. In: *Intracranial Tumours*. Thomas CC (ed). Springfield, IL: Thomas Books, 1932.
70. Bindal AK, Bindal RK, Hess KR, et al. Surgery versus radiosurgery in the treatment of brain metastasis. *J Neurosurg* 1996;84:748–754.
71. Brega K, Robinson WA, Winston K, et al. Surgical treatment of brain metastases in malignant melanoma. *Cancer* 1990;66:2105–2110.
72. Cabantog AM, Bernstein M. Complications of first craniotomy for intra-axial brain tumour. *Can J Neurol Sci* 1994;21:213–218.
73. Haar F, Patterson R. Surgery for metastatic intracranial neoplasm. *Cancer* 1972;30:1241–1245.
74. Vecht CJ, Haaxma-Reiche H, Noordijk EM, et al. Treatment of single brain metastasis: Radiotherapy alone or combined with neurosurgery? *Ann Neurol* 1993;33:583–590.

# 5

# Radiosurgery for Brain Metastases

Laurie E. Blach
Sammie Coy
Aizik Loft Wolf

The treatment of brain metastases in the past was "3,000 in 10" (3,000 cGy in 10 fractions) to the whole brain. It was, but no longer is, a "no brainer" (1). Today, with the development of radiosurgical techniques, this is not the case. Radiosurgery (RS) has been shown to be an effective, minimally invasive outpatient treatment option for brain metastases (2), and many patients with brain metastases are now treated with radiosurgery. However, few patients in the United States were treated with this technique prior to the 1990s. Therefore, for many oncologists, this area is a "black box". This chapter will attempt to bring light to this very highly sophisticated and complex technology.

The advances in the treatment of brain metastases with radiosurgery have improved patient outcomes, particularly for limited intracranial disease with controlled systemic disease (3). Previously, the development of brain metastases was a death sentence. Treatment with whole-brain radiation therapy (WBRT) alone resulted in a 4-6 month median survival with 50 percent of patients dying of neurological causes (4,5). With the addition of RS for treatment of brain metastases, this is no longer the case (6–8).

Stereotactic radiosurgery delivers high doses of radiation to small intracranial tumors while sparing the surrounding normal tissues and critical structures (2). Conventional external beam radiotherapy (EBRT) utilizes standard daily doses of 180 to 300 cGy per fraction given, for a total of approximately 3,000 to 8,000 cGy over 2 to 8 weeks. Radiosurgery delivers treatment in 1 to 5 fractions using doses of approximately 10 to 40 Gy. Table 5.1 illustrates the basic differences in EBRT and RS treatment. RS is a very exacting

TABLE 5.1 Comparison of EBRT and RS Characteristics

|  | EBRT | RADIOSURGERY |
|---|---|---|
| Dose | 180–200 cGy | 1,000–4,000 cGy |
| Fractions | 10-40 | 1-5 |
| Dose rate | 400 mu/min | 1,000 mu/min (Trilogy) |
| Time | 2–8 weeks | 1 day to 2 weeks |
| Margin | 0.5-2 cm | 0-0.2 cm |
| Treatment Accuracy | 0.3-1 cm | <1 mm–2 mm |
| Treatment Time per fraction | 5–20 min | 15 min-5 hours (avg. 1hour, 22 min) |

and precise treatment technique in which a tumor is ablated by very high doses of highly focused radiation.

Local control rates for radiosurgery in treating brain metastases are approximately 80–97 percent (2,9,10), while the morbidity and mortality are low. The benefits of RS as compared to surgery include minimally invasive techniques, reduction of hospitalization time and cots, excellent local tumor control rates (even in radioresistant oncotypes), and extremely low morbidity (6-10). Progression free survival (PFS) and median survival recurrence rates are comparable to results of surgery and radiation and better than those achieved with WBRT (9). RS also reduces the risk of neurological death (7-9).

The history of RS goes back to 1951 when Lars Leksell, a Swedish neurosurgeon, first described radiosurgery techniques. RS was developed as a surgical tool, by a neurosurgeon, hence the name radiosurgery. The modern concept of RS is based upon the Leksell stereotactic system in which multiple beams are fired from different points in multiple arcs while converging on a center tumor (Figure 5.1).

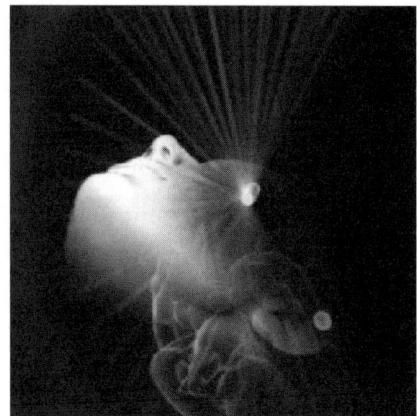

FIGURE 5.1   Multiple beams are fired from different points, converging on a target. (Used with permission Elekta, Stockholm, Sweden).

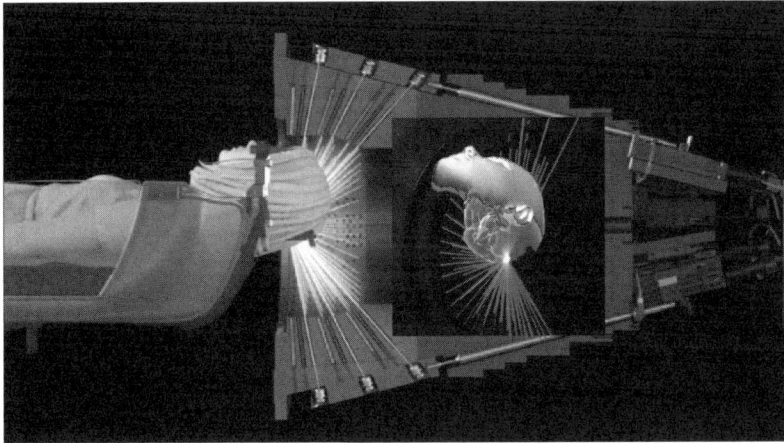

FIGURE 5.2 Gamma knife treatment unit that employs 201 cobalt sources converging on a point in space. (Used with permission Elekta, Stockholm, Sweden).

The radiation is spread throughout the brain so that only the tumor receives a significant dose of radiation. Regions just outside the target are exposed to zero, or one beam producing minimal radiation. The goal is to destroy an intracranial tumor by converging multiple beams on a targeted point, while minimizing radiation to the surrounding normal tissues and structures. Lars Leksell developed a gamma knife treatment unit that employs 201 Cobalt sources converging on a point in space (Figure 5.2). The earliest use of the gamma knife involved functional disorders. (Further discussion of specific disorders is beyond the scope of this chapter.)

The principles of stereotaxis using strict fixation and a specialized frame of reference have been widely adopted. For treatment with the gamma knife unit, a rigid external frame, the Leksell frame (Elekta, Stockholm, Sweden), is attached to the skull for immobilization (Figure 5.3). This provides a frame based coordinate system for positioning the frame so that the target is at the

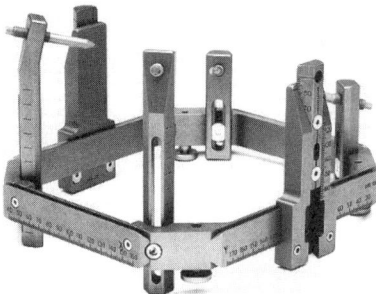

FIGURE 5.3 The Leksell frame (Elekta, Stockholm, Sweden) is attached to the skull for immobilization and provides a frame-based coordinate system for positioning the frame so that the target is at the beam isocenter. (Used with permission Elekta, Stockholm, Sweden).

beam isocenter (beam intersection point). One of the earliest gamma knife radiosurgery units (Elekta, Stockholm, Sweden) was the model U (Figure 5.4).

In the United States, the first gamma knife unit for serial production was installed in Pittsburgh, Pennsylvania, in 1987. In the 1990s gamma knife radiosurgery became accepted internationally through widespread dissemination of the technology and experience. The ability to utilize and incorporate magnetic resonance imaging (MRI) was a significant step in the advancement because tumors became more visible. Newer models, which incorporated knowledge gained and new developments in technology, were developed over time. The model C employs an automatic positioning system (APS) in which the target positions are reached automatically (Figure 5.5). Before this model was adopted for radiosurgery, all positioning was done by trunnion mode by hand, increasing the risk of human error and requiring timely QA[TSC1] procedures.

The newest gamma knife model is the Perfexion shown in Figure 5.6. This new system is fully automated and utilizes an automatic positioning system and an automatic helmet changer. These refinements will further reduce the chance of human error and speed treatment delivery times. The Perfexion will also allow easier treatment of base of skull and head and neck lesions.

Gamma knife radiosurgery (GKS) is the gold standard to which other delivery methods of RS are compared. There are approximately 250 gamma-

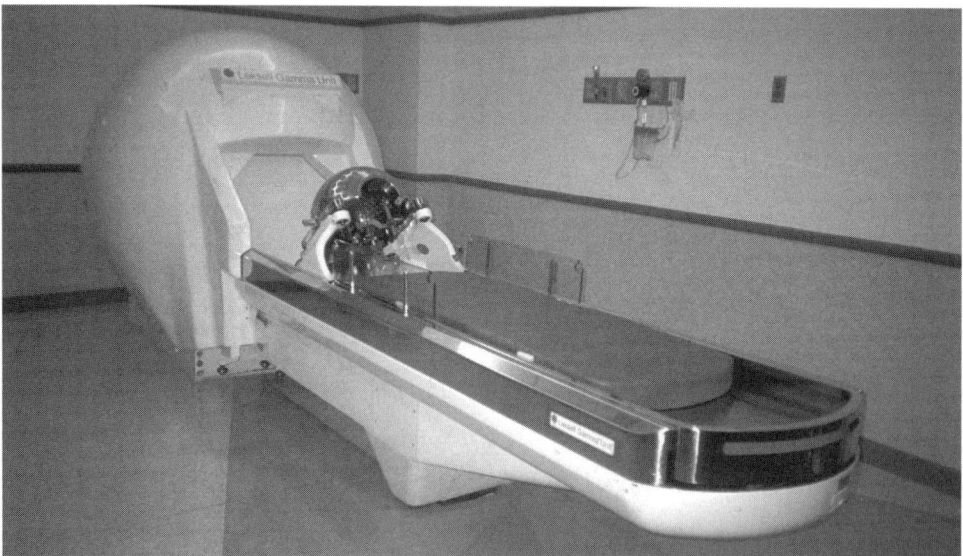

FIGURE 5.4   One of the earliest gamma knife radiosurgery units was the model U. (Used with permission Elekta, Stockholm, Sweden).

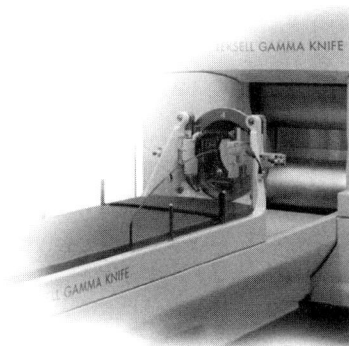

FIGURE 5.5 The gamma knife model C with automatic positioning system (APS).

knife units in use in 250 hospitals worldwide, 30 percent of which are in the United States. In fact, the longest and broadest experience with RS has been with the gamma knife system. As of December 2006, approximately 400,000 patients have been treated with the gamma knife system, more than 141,000 of which were treated for brain metastases.

Linac-based stereotactic systems were also developed to perform radiosurgery and have become competitive with the gamma knife system. Linac-based RS systems include the Trilogy, Varian Medical Systems, Inc. (Palo Alto, CA) CyberKnife (Accuray, Sunnyvale, CA), Novalis (BrainLAB, Feldkichen, Germany). TomoTherapy (Madison, WI) and Proton Therapy units can be added to the list of machines capable of delivering RS. A list of RS systems is displayed in Table 5.2. Later in the chapter, details and illustrations of these

TABLE 5.2 Radiosurgery Systems

Elekta Oncology Systems Ltd. (Stockholm, Sweden)

Novalis™ (BrainLAB, Feldkichen, Germany)

X-Knife™ Radionics, Inc. (Burlington, MA, USA)

Linear accelerator Scalpel™ (Zmed, Inc., Ashland, MA, USA)

Trilogy, Varian Medical Systems, Inc. (Palo Alto, CA, USA)

Nomos Corp. (Sewickley, PA, USA)

CyberKnife® (Accuray, Sunnyvale CA, USA)

TomoTherapy, Inc. (Madison, WI, USA)

Proton Therapy Systems

Optivus Technology, Inc. (San Benardino, CA, USA)

Ion Beam Applications (Lovain-la-Neuve, Belgium)

Varian Medical Systems, Inc. (Palo Alto, CA, USA)

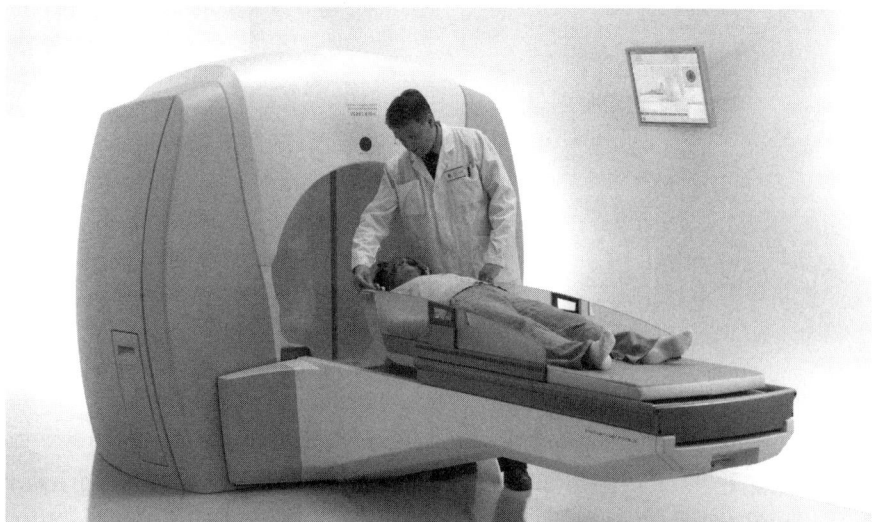

FIGURE 5.6    The Perfexion, the newest gamma knife radiosurgery system. (Used with permission Elekta, Stockholm, Sweden).

different systems are presented. All of these systems are able to provide local control of tumors in the brain without open surgery.

The Linac-based systems can utilize frame-based and/or frameless systems. Treatment can be delivered in 1 to 5 fractions with the frameless systems, whereas the frame-based systems deliver treatment in only 1 fraction. Both approaches have their benefits and proponents. Linac-based systems can also treat both cranial and extracranial targets. Extracranial radiosurgery is also referred to as "body radiosurgery" or "stereotactic body radiotherapy" (SBRT), but further discussion of SBRT is beyond the scope of this chapter.

Frameless, noninvasive RS methods were developed, which use dental molds or skeletal references and preclude the need for skeletal fixation (Figure 5.7). The frameless systems are less invasive than frame-based systems, but the stable alignment of the tumor with respect to the treatment isocenter is less certain. Some departments feel comfortable using only frame-based systems. Others rely on frame-based systems for tumors close to critical structures. On the other hand, with patients who are edentulous or uncooperative, the frameless systems can be unreliable. Most Linac RS systems utilize computed tomography (CT) for treatment planning. MRI can be fused to the CT system, but this introduces additional uncertainty and a component of human subjectivity.

The key benefit that all of these systems provide is a significant improvement in accuracy and precision (as low as 2 mm using frame-based fixation) when compared to standard external beam treatments. This allows for a sig-

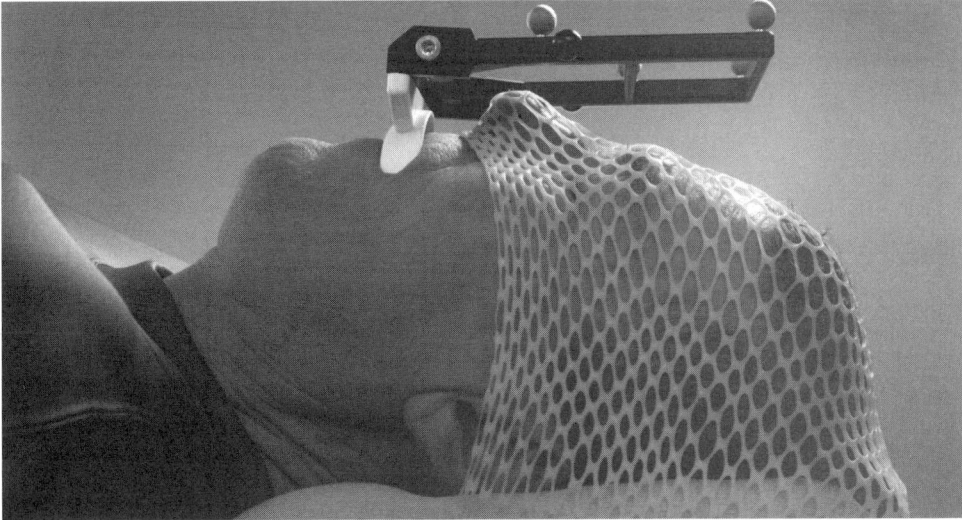

FIGURE 5.7    An example of a frameless system with mask and dental mold.

nificant reduction in the tumor margin, the normal brain tissue surrounding the tumor that is included in the treatment volume, which accounts for patient movement and/or set-up uncertainty. The reduction of treated volume reduces the risk of acute and long-term toxicity by reducing exposure of normal and critical brain structures to radiation.

## Indications for Radiosurgery

The current indications and uses of radiosurgery in the treatment of brain metastases is controversial and covered in great detail elsewhere in this book. However, the medical oncologist is often the first physician to see the patient after initial diagnoses of brain metastases or after the discovery of new or recurrent intracranial lesions. At that time, the first question is whether the patient is symptomatic. In the past, most patients with newly discovered brain metastases were routinely started on steroids. This is no longer the case. If the patient is asymptomatic and neuroimaging does not show significant edema or midline shift, there is an option not to begin using steroids. Referral to the radiation oncologist, neurosurgeon, or radiosurgery team then ensues. Patients who are severely symptomatic or present with a seizure are often admitted, evaluated, and treated on an in-patient basis. Some departments have coordinated radiosurgery clinics or tumor boards where cases are presented and discussed with the whole radiosurgery treatment team. Others have not. Each department, institution, or radiosurgery team develops its own indications for RS based upon available data, experience, availability of research protocols, and other criteria. These indications do change over time as new experience is acquired and new data becomes available.

## Multiple Metastases

Patients who have previously been treated with WBRT (a one-time-only treatment) for multiple metastases can be followed closely with follow up MRIs every 2 to 3 months. When new intracranial lesions develop or old ones grow, these patients can be referred for radiosurgery treatment. The purpose for this approach is to maintain local intracranial disease control, minimize resultant neurological symptomatology, and maintain quality of life.

The cut-off, or maximum number of intracranial metastases in a patient with newly diagnosed brain metastases that should receive RS, is controversial and an area of significant disagreement that continues to fluctuates over time. Many radiosurgical centers have historically set a predefined limit to the number of metastases that can be treated with RS. In the early 1990s this limit was often set at one to three brain tumors (9,11). Later that number was increased to four (12,13). More recently, that maximum number of brain metastases that are treated with RS has increased even further (14-18).

Previously it was impractical to treat more than 3 to 5 brain metastases on a nondedicated Linac-based machine as it had to be QA'd [TSC2] and adjusted for radiosurgery treatment at the end of each treatment day. Technically, the maximum number of lesions that can be treated with RS in a given day is influenced by a patient's ability to tolerate the treatment experience, the patient's Karnofsky performance status (KPS), and time constraints. Time constraints are influenced by treatment delivery time, technical efficiency of the treatment team, type of machine utilized for treatment, scheduling issues affecting a nondedicated RS machine, and rate of radiation delivery. Although it is possible to deliver treatment over 2 days to overcome some of these issues, this is rarely done.

With today's technology, such as the use of intensity modulated radiosurgery treatment and planning (IMRS), patients with 20 to 30 small brain tumors can be treated comfortably within the defined technical and patient-related time constraints (19). In addition, it was once thought that the number of brain metastases was a prognosticator for survival; therefore, patients with multiple brain metastases were expected to have a lower survival potential than that which now justifies the use of RS. According to Dr. Larson, "We're now seeing that the number of tumors is a poor predictor for how many other (tumors) may appear later, either in the brain or elsewhere in the body" (19).

There is some evidence that when numerous multiple lesions are treated with RS, the dose delivery is similar to whole-brain radiation therapy. However, the data suggests otherwise (15-18). Yang et al. showed that 50 percent of the brain volume receives less than 500 cGy and that the dose gradient is extremely steep (16). Figure 5.8 illustrates the whole-brain dose and isodose distribution of a patient treated with gamma knife RS to multiple lesions, 21 brain tumors treated over 2 treatment days. This illustrates that there is significant brain sparing even with the treatment of many multiple metastases. When evaluated, treatment of numerous metastases with radiosurgery alone is possible and safe (15-18).

The uninvolved brain is spared and receives significantly less than 6 Gy (white line). The pictures on page 116 show the patient's response to treatment. The patient later died of systemic disease progression, not because of brain metastases.

### Location and Shape of Metastases

Location of brain metastases close to the brain stem, critical, or radiosensitive structures does not, definitively, preclude the use of RS. The dose prescribed may be reduced, fractionated (20), or beam shaped to minimize dose to the critical structures. The University of California at San Francisco (UCSF) experience delivering gamma knife radiosurgery for brain-stem metastases showed excellent freedom from progression (FFP) with low morbidity when using a dose of 16 Gy (21). The findings were similar to those of others researchers (22-24). Figure 5.9 illustrates RS treatment of a metastases to the brainstem and resultant response. Cystic or hemorrhagic metastases may benefit from stereotactic aspiration with RS to the residual nodular component.

## Radiosurgery Planning

The hallmark of RS treatment planning and delivery is that it minimizes radiation to the surrounding normal tissues while delivering the desired dose to tumor volume. This is achieved by a steep dose fall-off beyond the metastases and a conformal dose plan. Dose conformality is measured by dividing the volume within the prescription isodose line by the target volume. This results in the conformity factor. The ideal conformity factor is one, meaning that the volume receiving the full dose is equal to the tumor volume. A conformity factor of less than one suggests that a part of the metastases is not within the prescribed treatment area. Acceptable conformity factors range from approxi-

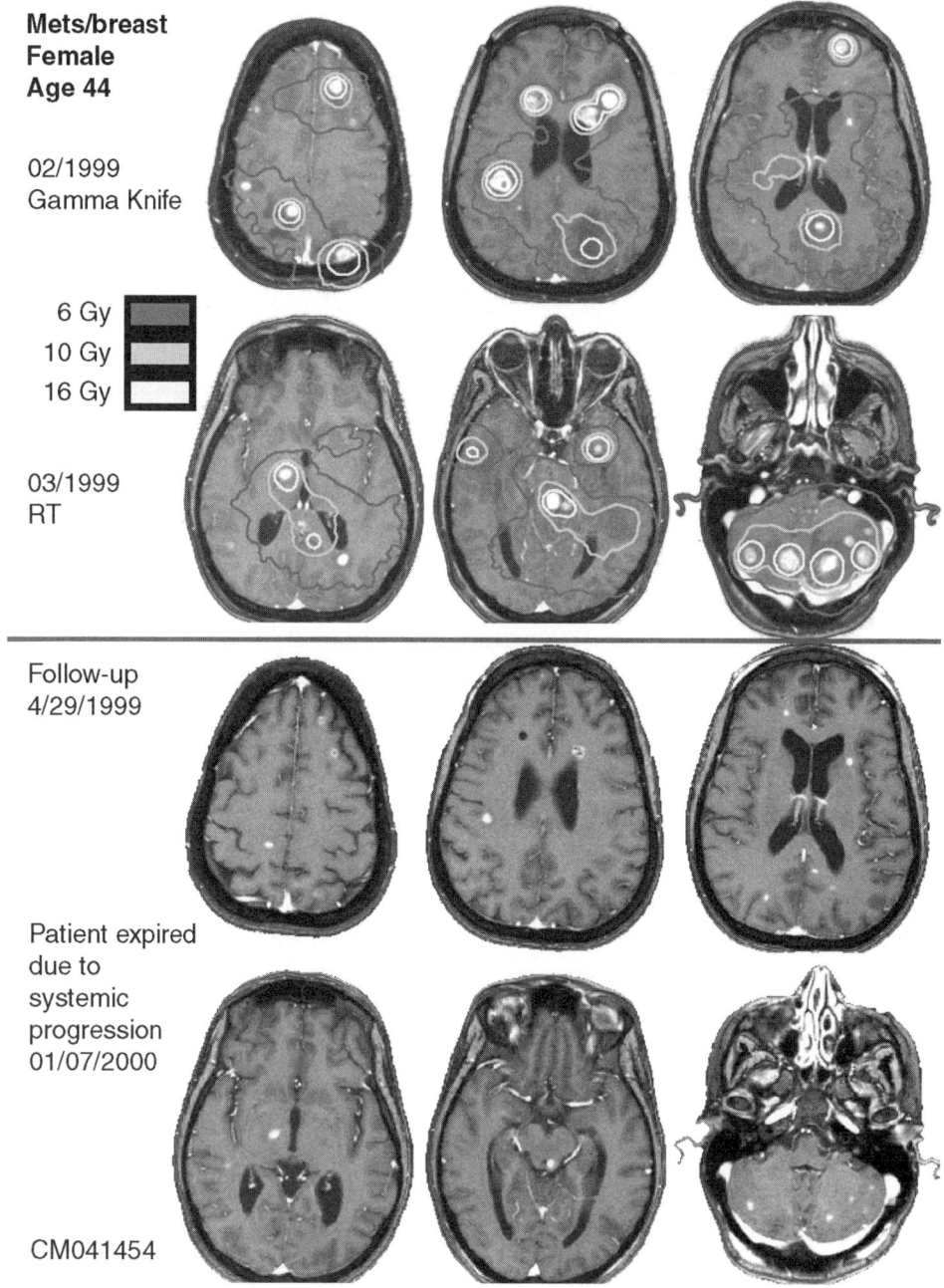

**Mets/breast
Female
Age 44**

02/1999
Gamma Knife

6 Gy
10 Gy
16 Gy

03/1999
RT

Follow-up
4/29/1999

Patient expired
due to
systemic
progression
01/07/2000

CM041454

FIGURE 5.8    A patient treated with multiple brain metastases to 16 Gy (the white line).

**Mets/Breast**
**Female**
**Age 46**

Brain stem lesion shown

Day of Tx

1.5 Month
Follow-up

3.5 Month
Follow-up

No previous RT
3 sites Tx'd

16 Gy

06 Gy

DL100150

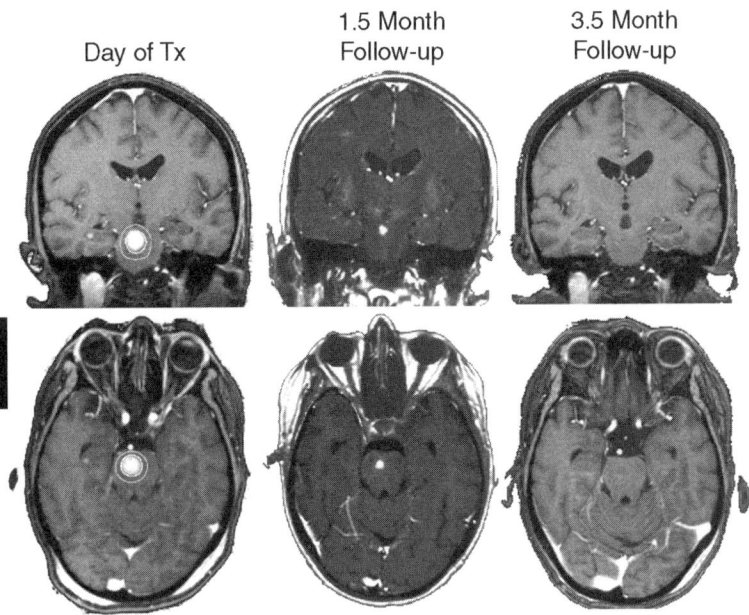

FIGURE 5.9   RS treatment of a metastases to the brain stem and resultant response at 1.5 and 3.4 months. 16 Gy (white line) was prescribed to the 50 percent isodose line. The 6 Gy line (grey) shows the rapid dose fall-off outside the prescription line.

mately 1–1.2. Dose conformality is an objective way to compare different plans, the goal being to reduce the amount of tissue outside of the metastases receiving full dose.

## Available Radiosurgery Technology

The remaining chapter attempts to describe in great detail different radiosurgery machines and their treatment procedures with respect to brain metastases. The purpose of this chapter is to familiarize the reader with radiosurgery and the different methods of treatment delivery. The authors are gamma knife users and, as such, are biased toward this technology. However, this chapter is not intended to advocate one system over another (Table 5.3).

### Gamma Knife Radiosurgery

Gamma knife surgery represents a major advance in available treatment options for patients with brain metastases. With radiosurgery, a surgical inci-

TABLE 5.3 Comparison of Gamma Knife and Linear Accelerator Radiosugery Machines

| MACHINE | GAMMA KNIFE | LINAC-BASED |
| --- | --- | --- |
| Immobilization | Frame-based | Frame based or Frameless (CyberKnife/Frameless) |
| Imaging | MRI | CT with MRI fusion available |
| Radiation delivery | 201 fixed concentric nonopposed beams | Nonco-planar arcs/IMRS/IMRT |
| Radiation Planning | Shot packing planning | Shot packing with cone based arc delivery or IMRT/IMRS planning and delivery |
| Radiation Source | 201 cobalt 60 sources | Linear Accelerator (6 MV Photons) |
| Collimators | 4, 8, 14, 18 mm | Circular Cone Based/MLC |
| Radiation Tx Delivery | Gamma knife unit | Trilogy/CyberKnife/TomoTherapy/ Modified Linac |
| Treatment Date | Same day | Same day or delayed day |
| Fractions | One | 1 to 5 |
| Sites | Cranial only (Perfexion allows H&N tx) | Intracranial and extracranial |

sion is not required. The attendant risks of open neurosurgical procedures and anesthesia (hemorrhage, infection, cerebrospinal fluid leakage, etc.) are therefore avoided. The "blades" of the gamma knife are the 201 beams of cobalt radiation. Each portion of the target is positioned at the fixed intersection point of those beams (Figure 5.10).

The gamma knife system is the gold standard to which all other systems are compared. A rigid external frame, the Leksell frame (Elekta, Stockholm,

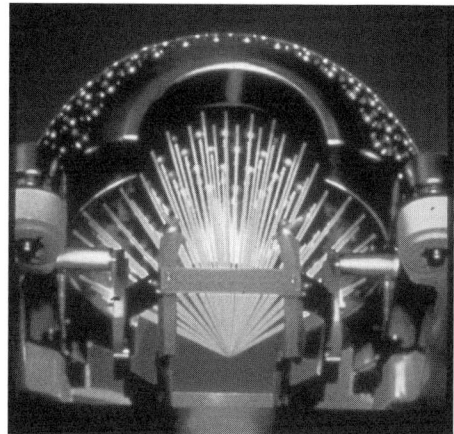

FIGURE 5.10 Gamma knife radiosurgery with 201 cobalt beams converging on a fixed point in space.

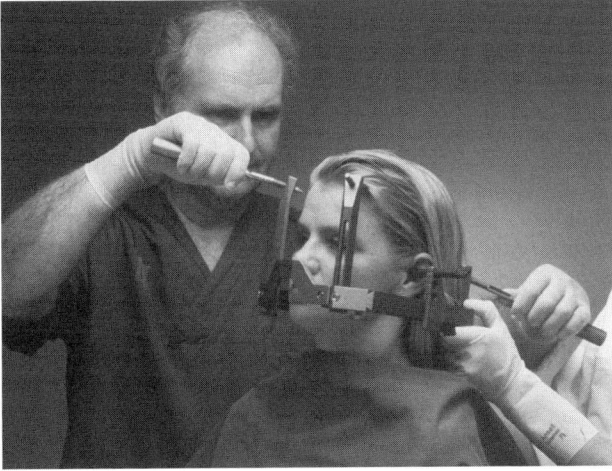

FIGURE 5.11 The placement of the Leksell frame for gamma knife radiosurgery. (Used with permission Elekta, Stockholm, Sweden).

Sweden), is attached to the skull for target and patient immobilization (Figure 5.11). A frame-based coordinate system, used for aligning the target and beam isocenter, is established by attaching an image localizer box to the Leksell frame prior to imaging. An MRI is then obtained for stereotactic localization. If needed, a stereotactic biopsy can be obtained at this juncture (Figure 5.12).

A treatment plan is developed using single or multiple isocenter shots with the Leksell Gamma Plan. The use of multiple isocenters (treatment positions) is referred to as shot packing or sphere packing (Figure 5.13).

Four collimator helmets are used interchangeably for gamma knife treatment, producing 4, 8, 14, and 18 mm beam sizes, respectively (Figure 5.14).

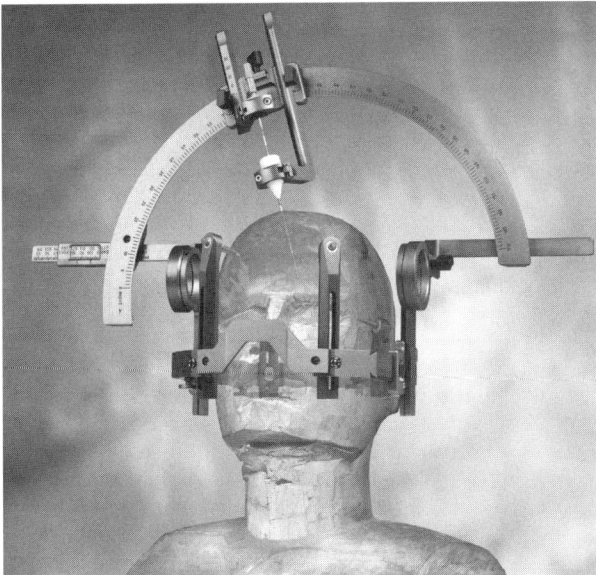

FIGURE 5.12 A stereotactic guided biopsy procedure using the Leksell frame

FIGURE 5.13 Shot packing to produce complete tumor coverage. The column on the left shows isocenter or shot placement in white. The column on the right shows the resultant dose distribution. The treatment is prescribed to a minimum dose of 12 Gy (shown in white). The 8 Gy line (in grey) shows significant rapid fall-off of the dose. A 5 month follow-up post treatment is shown at right.

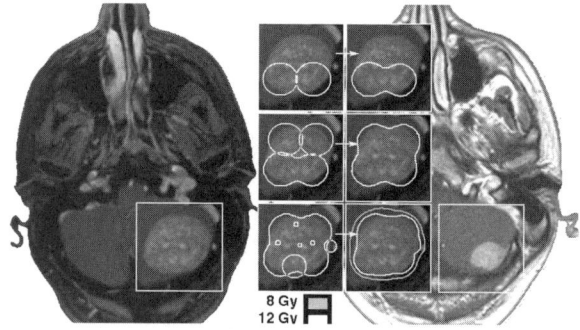

The Perfexion, the newest gamma knife model, has three beam size options, replacing 14 and 18 mm beam size with a 16 mm beam channel. A single 4 mm shot creates a 0.09 cubic centimeter (cc) treatment volume with a maximum dose range of 50 to 100. The 8, 14, and 18 mm collimator helmets result in larger treatment volumes when utilized (Table 5.4). However, multiple isocenter plans can be developed to conform to different tumor shapes and sizes A plugging pattern, the blocking of selected beams, can be added to further shape the dose distribution as needed to spare surrounding normal or critical structures. The treatment planning process for brain metastases takes on average 1 hour (range 5 minutes to 2 hours or more). The gamma knife treatment is delivered the same day the plan is completed.

Gamma knife target volumes generally receive a dose range of 50 to 100 percent of the maximum dose (the 50 percent isodose line encompasses the target volume). There is rapid dose fall off as you go into the surrounding normal tissue (outside the 50 percent isodose line). For Linac-based systems, the prescription line is usually to the 80 percent isodose line. The possible advantage of dose inhomogeneity inherent to the gamma knife plan over dose uniformity, in a Linac-based plan, may account for the reported higher local control rates with gamma knife radiosurgery reported in a 2007 Radiation Therapy Oncology Group (RTOG) study (25).

TABLE 5.4 Collimator Helmet Single Isocenter Shot Delivery and Resultant Volume Receiving at Least 50 Percent of Maximum Dose by Helmet Size (approximate)

| Collimator helmet size | Resultant volume |
| --- | --- |
| 4 mm | 0.09 cc |
| 8 mm | 0.6 cc |
| 14 mm | 2.9 cc |
| 18 mm | 5.8 cc |

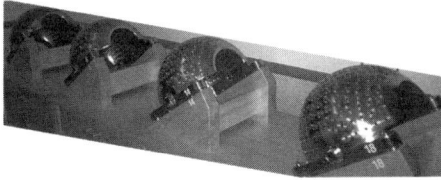

FIGURE 5.14  Four model U gamma knife radiosurgery collimator helmets produce 4, 8, 14, and 18mm beam sizes. They are changed manually between treatment shots as needed.

Table 5.5 describes the procedural steps of gamma knife radiosurgery accomplished during one treatment day. The neurosurgeon, and often the radiation oncologist, must see the patient in consultation prior to the procedure date.

Each gamma knife department has its own specific protocols. In our department, conscious sedation is utilized for frame placement in our Gamma Knife Neurosurgery Suite. Some departments do not use conscious sedation and some place the frame in the operating room (OR) or recovery room (RR). Treatment planning is performed by the physicist with the input of the neurosurgeon and radiation oncologist. It is a team effort. The time of delivery of the gamma knife treatment varies, depending upon number of lesions treated, dose delivered, and age of cobalt sources. It can range from less than one-half hour, for a single isocenter shot for a single metastatic lesion, to more than 3 hours for multiple metastases. The dose and duration of Decadron on which the patient is sent home varies, depending on whether the patient is symptomatic or already on Decadron.

The MRI technique utilized at the time of gamma knife radiosurgery varies from institution to institution. The authors utilize a high resolution triple con-

TABLE 5.5  Gamma Knife Radiosurgery Procedure

Pretreatment antibiotics and Decadron

Conscious sedation

Local anesthesia applied to pin sites

Application of Leksell head frame

Placement of MRI localizer box

MRI thin cuts, triple contrast

Treatment planning

Gamma knife treatment

Removal of frame

Pin sites cleaned and dressed

Posttreatment Decadron administered

Pt sent home on Decadron for 10 days w/GI prophylaxis

trast MRI scan with 1 mm cuts. New, previously undetected metastases are often found during RS planning. Reports in the literature show that this happens in up to 50 percent of cases, depending upon the MRI protocol and dose of contrast utilized at the time of RS planning (26,27). Other centers use the same MRI protocol for primary tumor imaging as they do for RS treatment planning and are thus unlikely to have the same results. Each center develops its own approach.

## Linac-Based Systems

Linac is short for the term linear accelerator. Linac machines may be dedicated or nondedicated. Nondedicated Linac machines may be used for conventional radiation therapy and radiosurgery treatment delivery. Linac-based RS machines can deliver treatments over one to several days, yielding a flexibility that is not available with GKS. Treatments that are given over time are referred to as fractionated stereotactic radiotherapy (FSR) or stereotactic radiotherapy (SRT). The linear accelerator based machines utilize a cone-based arc system and/or an intensity modulated radiotherapy (IMRT) based treatment planning and delivery technique.

*Trilogy image-guided radiosurgery system*    The Trilogy image guided radiosurgery system (Varian, Palo Alto, CA) is one of the newer Linac-based radiosurgery systems (Figure 5.15). The Trilogy machine functions both as a Linac system for external beam radiotherapy (EBRT) and as radiosurgery. It is manufactured by Varian, which supplies a majority of the radiation therapy treatment machines in the United States. The Trilogy machine combines imaging and treatment in one machine. It provides digital image guidance both for radiotherapy and radiosurgery, using 2D, 3D CT, and fluoroscopic imaging for patient positioning and robotic guidance. The digitally reconstructed images (DRRs) from the simulator are transferred to the treatment machine. The images obtained on the Trilogy unit are then overlaid and compared to DRRs. The Trilogy machine records the necessary shifts for accurate set-up. The patient is then moved robotically into the exact desired treatment position.

The Trilogy system has both frame-based and frameless RS applications. The frame-based system is similar to others and, in addition, has an optical tacking system attached (Figure 5.16). The frame is placed prior to simulation. The frameless system utilizes a dental bite block, an optical tracking system, and a head mask (Figures 5.17 and 5.18).

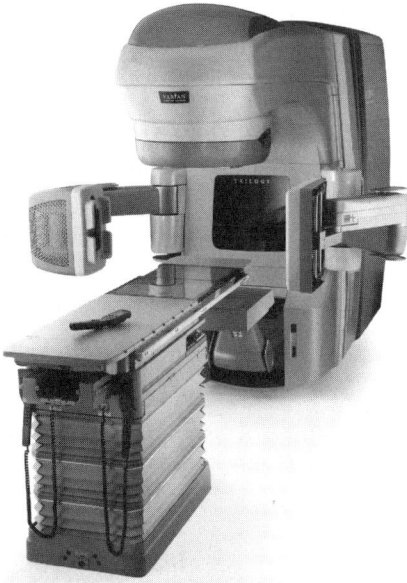

FIGURE 5.15   The Trilogy image guided radiosurgery machine. (Used with permission of Varian, Palo Alto, CA).

The Trilogy system utilizes a dose rate of 1000mu/min for RS treatments. During regular EBRT treatment, the dose is delivered at approximately 400 mu/min. This increases the dose delivery rate and significantly reduces the actual treatment time when compared to other Linac-based systems.

Optical camera tracking technology continually checks the patient's position as the treatment proceeds. The combined system can detect if and when the patient or targeted area is out of position, determine exactly how much the patient must be moved to put the tumor squarely into the path of the treatment beam (Figure 5.19).

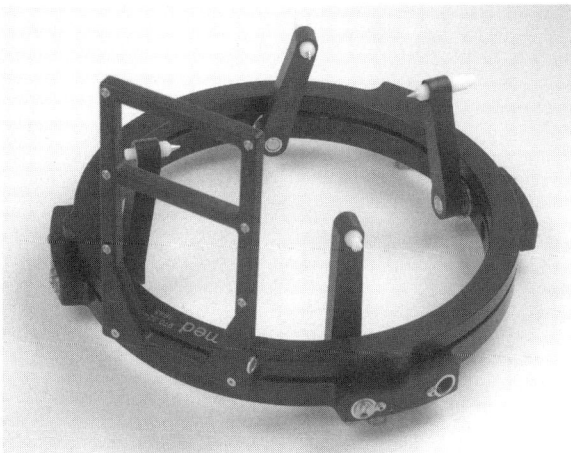

FIGURE 5.16    Frame-based system for RS delivery with optical guidance. (Used with permission of Varian, Palo Alto, CA).

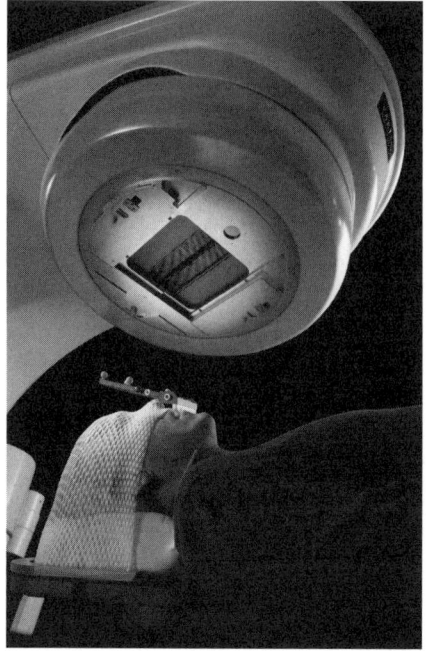

FIGURE 5.17 Trilogy frameless radiosurgery treatment set-up with mask, bite block, and optical tracking. (Used with permission of Varian, Palo Alto, CA).

The Trilogy system facilitates planning radiosurgery delivery with two different planning systems (Figures 5.20 and 5.21). Radiosurgery can be delivered using a cone-based system similar to other Linac-based radiosurgery systems (such as Z-Med or Brain Lab) or by using intensity modulated radiotherapy (IMRT) planning and delivery techniques. The cone-based planning system is similar to the gamma knife planning system in that it uses shot packing; however, treatment is delivered with arcs. Various cone sizes, which are affixed to the treatment head for RS, are available. The use of IMRT planning and delivery techniques for radiosurgery is called intensity modulated radiosurgery (IMRS). As with IMRT for external beam treatment delivery, dynamic sliding mutileaf collimators (MLCs) are utilized. The IMRS system allows for faster

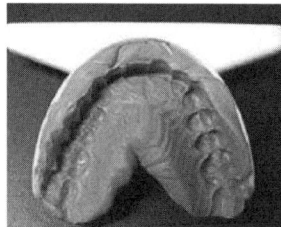

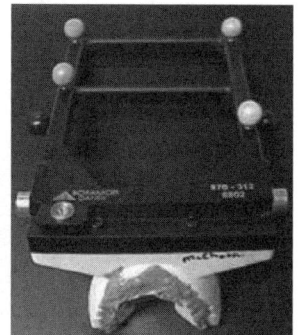

FIGURE 5.18 The dental mold and optical tracking system attachment is shown above. (Used with permission of Varian, Palo Alto, CA).

FIGURE 5.19 The optical tracking system that accounts and corrects for patient movement during treatment. (Used with permission of Varian, Palo Alto, CA).

planning and treatment delivery than the cone-based system in situations where many isocenter shots are needed, such as for multiple metastases, larger and nonspherical lesions, or for dose sculpting around vital or critical structures (Table 5.6).

*The CyberKnife System*    The CyberKnife system (Accuray, Inc., Sunnyvale, California) utilizes a condensed linear accelerator mounted on a robotic arm (Figures 5.22 and 5.23). The CyberKnife system monitors internal reference points, anatomy, or implanted fiducial markers, and corrects for patient movement real time during treatment (Figure 5.24). Treatment planning and delivery is based upon computed tomography (CT) imaging. Normal and critical structures are identified and contoured. Prescription dose and dose constraints are given for normal and critical structures. The treatment planning system utilizes an optimization algorithm, which identifies a set of beams that achieve an optimal dose distribution for a given patient (Figures 5.25 and 5.26). The CyberKnife radiosurgery treatment procedure is similar to that of the Trilogy frameless system (Table 5.6).

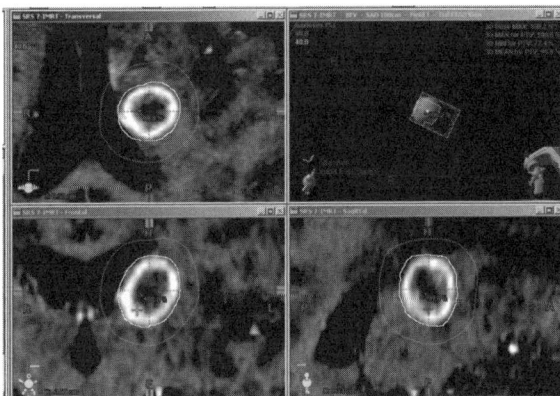

FIGURE 5.20 Eclipse IMRT plan for treatment of a solitary brain tumor. (Used with permission of Varian, Palo Alto, CA).

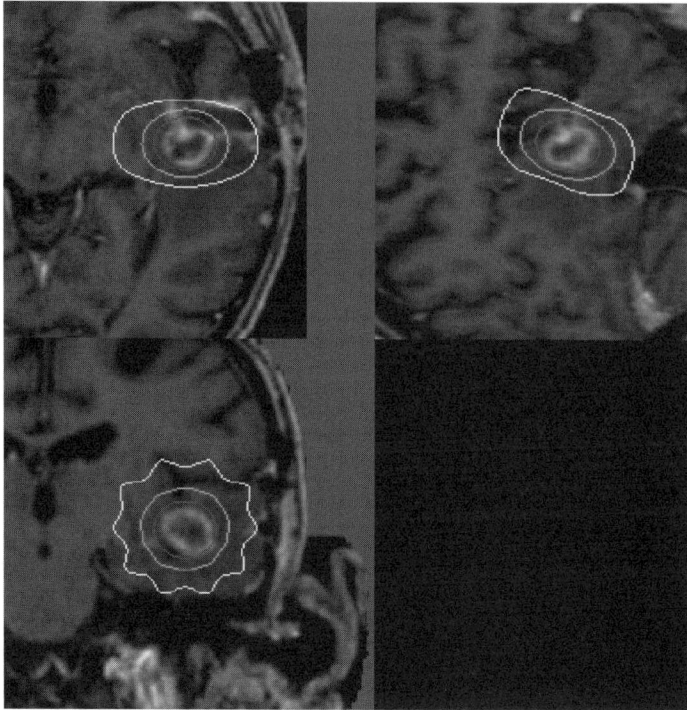

FIGURE 5.21    Cone-based treatment plan for a solitary brain tumor. (Used with permission of Varian, Palo Alto, CA).

*TomoTherapy* The TomoTherapy treatment system was designed in the 1990s. The goal was to develop a machine that was historically different, using advances in computing, imaging, and treatment delivery technologies. The machine looks like a CT scanner because it is based upon a CT scanner design (Figure 5.27). TomoTherapy uses integrated CT imaging to guide treatment, and the ring gantry design allows for helical 360° treatment delivery (Figure

TABLE 5.6  Procedure of Trilogy Radiosurgery

| FRAME-BASED | FRAMELESS |
| --- | --- |
| MRI obtained prior to treatment day | MRI obtained prior to treatment day |
| Frame placed in OR, office, or recovery room | Dental tray development and testing preformed |
| CT Simulation | CT Simulation performed; mask made |
| Treatment Planning | Treatment planning |
| Treatment on Trilogy unit that day | All above is done prior to treatment day and treatment on Trilogy unit in 1 to 5 fractions |
| Optical guidance utilized | Optical guidance utilized<br>IGRT with KV & cone beam available |

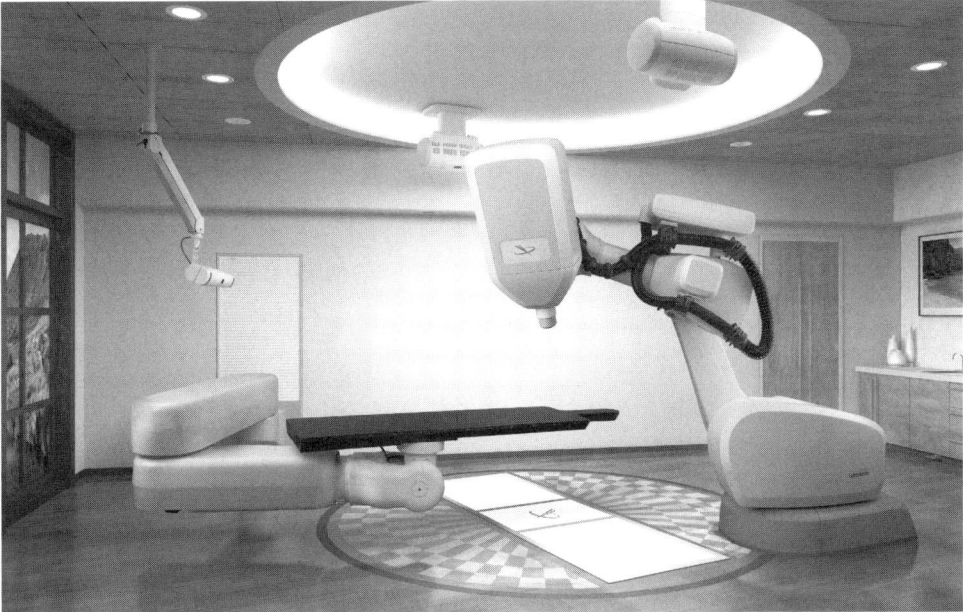

FIGURE 5.22    The CyberKnife System. (Used with permission of Accuray, Sunnyvale, CA).

5.28). TomoTherapy combines image guidance and intensity modulated radiation therapy (IGRT/IMRT) and adaptive planning. The IGRT/IMRT component of the technology can be used for radiosurgery and EBRT/IMRT treatment planning and delivery. Adaptive planning is less important for single fraction radiosurgery treatments than for multiple fraction treatment delivery. The

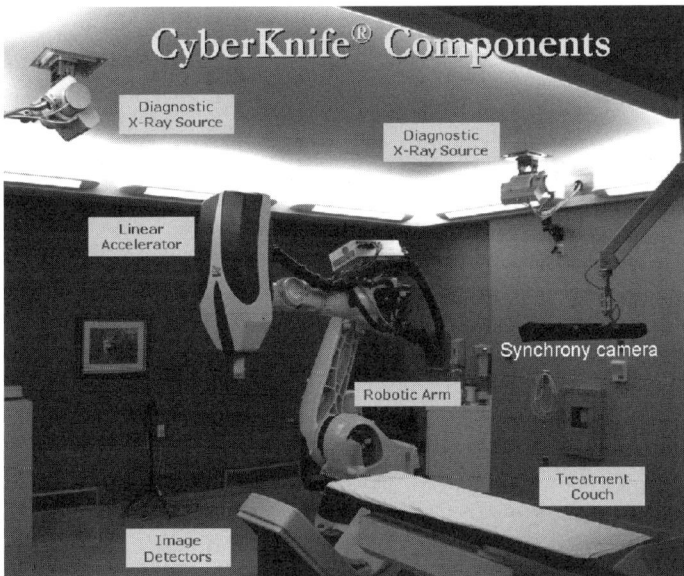

FIGURE 5.23 Cyber-Knife components. (Used with permission of Accuray, Sunnyvale, CA).

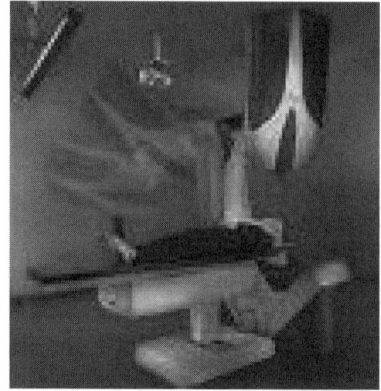

FIGURE 5.24 CyberKnife robotic arm moves during treatment. (Used with permission of Accuray, Sunnyvale, CA).

TomoTherapy radiosurgery treatment procedure is similar to that of the Trilogy frameless system (Table 5.6).

*Protons* The particle/proton beam currently exists in only a handful of centers in the United States. In addition to brain tumors, it treats body cancers in a fractionated manner. Due to the cost of the particle beam facility (>$100 million), little research on this system is currently available. However, an increasing number of proton facilities are being built around the country.

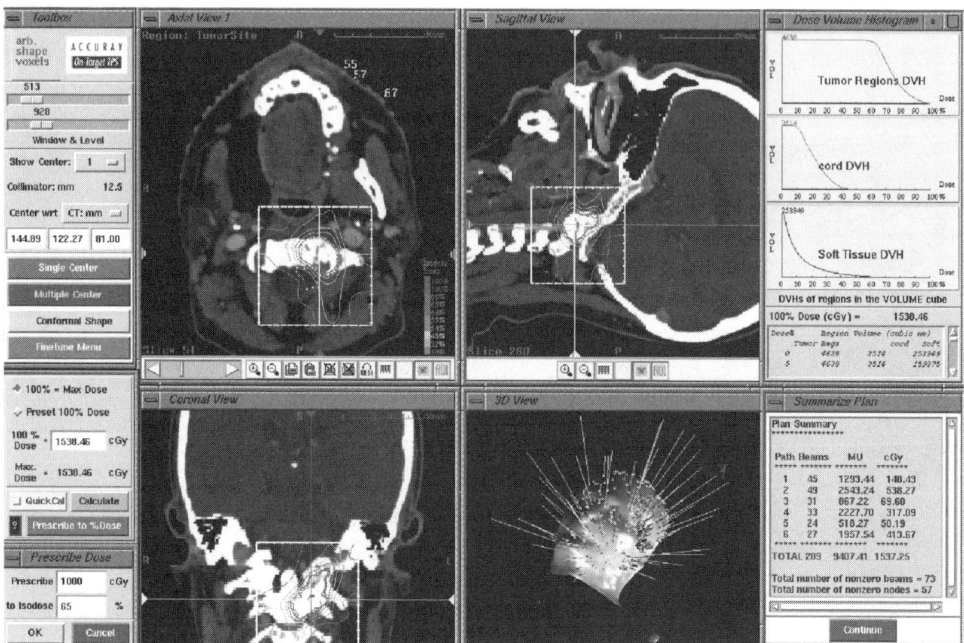

FIGURE 5.25 CyberKnife treatment planning system. (Used with permission of Accuray, Sunnyvale, CA).

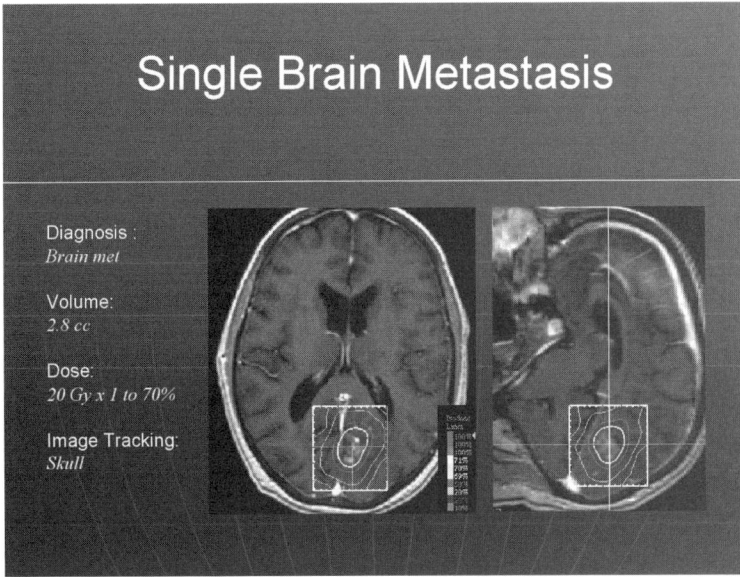

FIGURE 5.26   CyberKnife treatment plan for solitary brain tumor. (Used with permission of Accuray, Sunnyvale, CA).

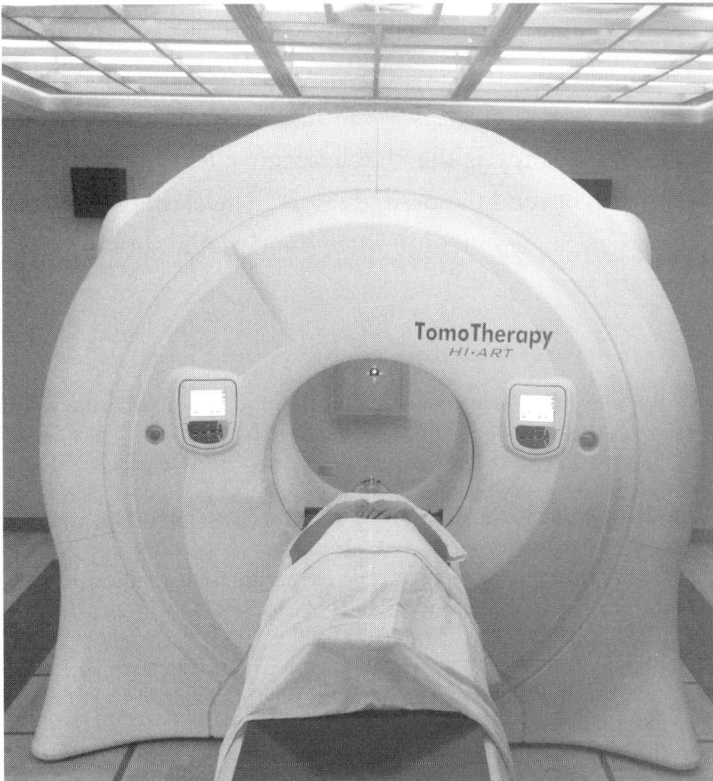

FIGURE 5.27   TomoTherapy machine looks like a CT scanner. (Used with permission of Tomotherapy, Inc., Madison, WI).

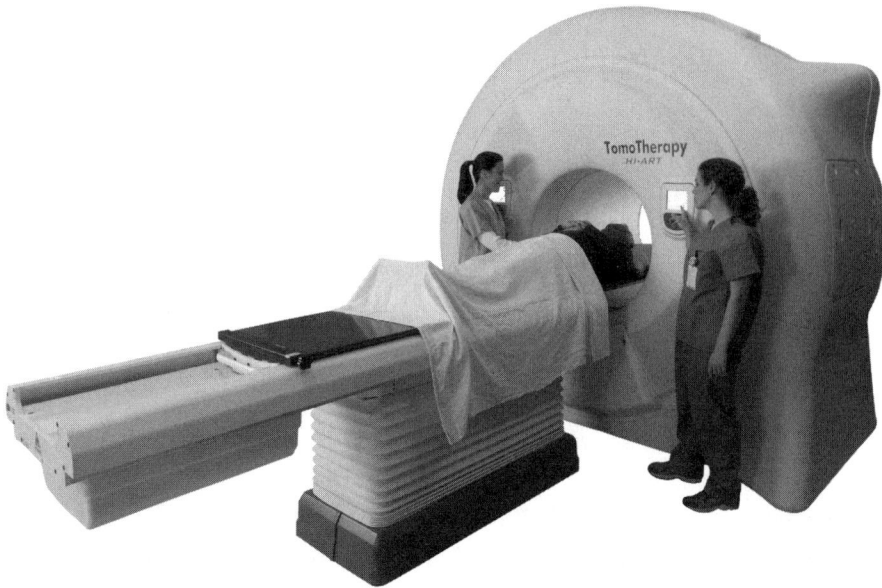

FIGURE 5.28    Tomotherapy Hi-ART Machine. (Used with permission of TomoTherapy, Inc., Madison, WI).

A proton is a stable particle with a positive charge equal to the negative charge of an electron. A proton's favorable absorption characteristics result from its charge and heavy mass, which is 1,835 times that of an electron. The major advantage of proton therapy is the characteristic energy distribution, in which the beam does not go beyond the desired target. The characteristic energy distribution of protons can be deposited in three-dimensional tumor locations.

## References

1. Shaw, EG. Radiotherapeutic management of multiple brain metastases: "3000 IN 10" whole brain radiation is no longer a "No Brainer." *Int J Radiat Oncol Biol Phys* 199;45: 253-254.
2. Alexander E, Moriarty TM, Davis RB, et al. *J of the NCI* 1995;87:34-39.
3. Lutterbach J, Bartelt S, Ostertag C. Long-term survival in patients with brain metastases. *J Cancer Res Clin Oncol* 2002;128: 417-425.
4. Gaspar L, Scott C, Rotman M, et al. Recursive partitioning analysis (RPA) of prognostic factors in three Radioation Therapy Oncology Group (RTOG) brain metastases trials. *Int J Radiat Oncolo Biol Phys* 1997;37:745-751.
5. Bogelt B, Gelber R, Kramer S, et al. The palliation of brain metastases: Final results of the first two studies by the Radiation Therapy Oncology Group (RTOG). *Int J Radiat Oncol Biol Phys* 1980;6:1-9.
6. Amendola BE, Wolf AL, Coy SR, et al. Brain metastases in renal cell carcinoma; management with Gamma Knife radiosurgery. *Cancer J* 2000;6:372-376.
7. Flickinger JC. Radiotherapy and radiosurgical management of brain metastases. *Curr Oncol Rep* 2001;3:484-489.

8.  Kondziolka D, Lunsford LD, Flickinger JC. Controversies in the management of multiple brain metastases: The roles of radiosurgery and radiation therapy. *Forum (Genova)* 2001;11:47-58.

9.  Gerosa M, Nicolato A, Foroni R, et al. Gamma knife radiosurgery for brain metastases: A primary therapeutic option. *J Neurosurg* (Suppl 5) 2002;97:515-524.

10. Mingione V, Oliveira M, Prasad D, et al. Gamma knife radiosurgery for melanoma metastases in the brain. *J Neurosurg* 2002;96:544-551.

11. Andrews DW, Scott CB, Sperduto, et al. Whole brain radiation therapy with or without stereotactic radiosurgery boost for patients with one to three brain metastases: Phase III results of the RTIG 9508 randomised trial. *Lancet* 2004;363:1665-1672.

12. Kondziolka D, Patel A, Lunsford LD, et al. Stereotactic radiosurgery plus whole brain radiotherapy verses radiotherapy alone for patients with multiple brain metastases. *Int J Radiat Oncol Biol Phys* 1999;45;427-434.

13. Aoyama H, Shirato H, Tago M, et al. Stereotactic radiosurgery plus whole-brain radiation therapy versus stereotactic radiosurgery alone for treatment of brain metastases: A randomized controlled trial. *JAMA* 2006;295:2483-2491.

14. J.L. Fox, M. Wharam, D. Rigamonti, et al. Can whole brain radiation be omitted in patients receiving radiosurgery for solitary or multiple brain metastases? *Int J Radiat Oncol Biol Phys* 2006;66:3, S251-S252.

15. Yamamoto M, Mitsunobu I, Shin-ichi N, et al. Gamma knife radiosurgery for numerous brain metastases: Is this safe? *Int J Radiat Oncol Biol Phys* 2002;53:279-1283.

16. Yang CCJ, Ting J, Wu X, et al. Dose volume histogram analysis of the gamma knife radiosurgery treating twenty-five metastatic intracranial tumors. *Stereotact Funct Neurosurg* 1998;70(Suppl.):41-49.

17. Yamamoto M, Ide M, Sakae O, et al. Gamma knife radiosurgery for ten or more brain metastases: Treatment results. Presented at the 5th International Stereotactic Radiosurgery Society Congress. June 10-13, 2001, Las Vegas [Abstract, p. 39].

18. Suzuki S, Omagari J, Nishio S, et al. Gamma knife radiosurgery for simultaneous multiple metastatic tumors. *J Neurosurg* 2000;93(Suppl 3):30-31.

19. Guralnick, E. Search, National Brain tumor Foundation Newsletter. Summer,2007;72:1-2.

20. Pahm CJ, Chang SD, Gibbs IC, et al. Preliminary visual field preservation after staged CyberKnife radiosurgery for perioptic lesions. *Neurosurgery* 2004;54:799-810.

21. Kased N, Huang K, Nakamura JL, et al. Gamma knife experience for brainstem metastases: the UCSF experience. *J Neruooncol* 2007;S11060-007:9458-64.

22. Fuentes S, Delsanti C, Metellus P, et al. Brainstem metastases: Management using gamma knife radiosurgery. *Neurosurgery* 200658:37-42

23. Huang CF, Kondziolka D, Flickinger JC, et al. Stereotactic radiosurgery for brainstem metastases. *J Neurosurgery* 1999;91:563—568.

24. Hussain A, Brown PD, Stafford SL, et al. Stereotactic radiosurgery for brainstem metastases: Survival, tumor control, and patient outcomes. *Int J Radiat Oncol Biol Phys* 2007; 67:521-524.

25. Shaw E, Scott C, Souhami L, et al. Single dose radiosurgical treatment of recurrent previously irradiated primary brain tumors and brain metastases: Final report of RTOG protocol 90-05. *Int J Radiant Oncol Biol Phys* 2000;47:291-298.

26. Engh, JA, Flickinger, JC, Niranjan, A, et al. Optimizing intracranial metastasis detection for stereotactic radiosurgery. *Stereotactic and Functional Neurosurgery* 2007;85:162-168.

27. Donahue BR, Goldberg JD, Golfinos JG, et al. Importance of MR technique for stereotactic radiosurgery. *Neurooncology* 2003;5:268-274.

# 6

# The Role of Targeted Therapy Without Whole-Brain Radiotherapy

Lawrence R. Kleinberg
Daniele Rigamonti

Until recently, whole-brain radiotherapy (WBRT) has been considered essential for all patients undergoing therapy of brain metastasis. This approach developed at a time when advanced imaging was not yet available and lesions, even if limited in number, could not be individually targeted. Treating the whole brain was the most rational approach to a situation where multiple lesions were often present and not possible to localize, where new metastasis could not be reliably detected until they had grown relatively large, and where good treatment options would not then be available.

Technologic developments, including ever higher resolution magnetic resonance imaging (MRI) scans and precise stereotactic treatment technology, have provided the opportunity to challenge the assumption that whole-brain radiotherapy is the optimal therapy for brain metastasis. It is now possible to detect and precisely treat individual lesions even as small as 2–3 mm, and patients can be closely followed with the goal of later treatment of any progression of subclinical disease before it is a threat. For many patients, it appears no longer to be necessary to prophylactically treat the whole brain, and it can be an appropriate choice to proceed with close follow-up after focal therapy and additional treatment only if needed.

The data summarized below suggest that many patients with a limited numbers of lesions, often up to 4 or more, which are detectable on MRI scanning can be appropriately treated with focal technologies without any demonstrable decrease in survival and with maintenance of good quality of life. Although large randomized trials assaying to definitively demonstrate equivalence have not been completed, retrospective and prospective data suggests that there is little or no difference in survival outcome although whole-brain radiotherapy significantly reduces the incidence of later brain metastasis.

The important issues to be considered by individual patients are summarized below. These include lack of survival benefit; toxicities; time commitment; likely need for future repeated treatment; need for prompt resumption of systemic therapies; risks of brain injury resulting from recurrence; number of metastasis; prognosis from systemic cancer, bulk of central nervous system (CNS) metastatic lesions; and individual views of the trade-off between the risks of brain tumor recurrence and treatment toxicities. In metastatic cancer where long-term survival is unlikely and cure rarely possible, it is appropriate for patients and physicians to carefully consider quality of life costs of whole-brain radiotherapy, even if there may be an as yet unappreciated modest survival advantage for those patients whose life expectancy is limited to the short or medium term. The exploration of this new approach for patients with limited brain metastasis was motivated by the desire of patients and oncologists to avoid the toxicities of whole-brain radiotherapy and prevent radiation-related interruptions of other needed treatments.

## Adjuvant Whole Brain Radiotherapy: Reduced Brain Recurrence but No Evidence of Survival Benefit

The available data has not suggested a meaningful survival benefit when whole-brain radiotherapy (WBRT) is added to localized therapies for brain metastasis even though there is a benefit in reduced distant brain tumor recurrence. This provides the justification for offering this choice to appropriately selected patients. Based on first principals, the addition of whole-brain radiotherapy to focal therapies of gross lesions is of potential survival benefit to only a limited proportion of patients. Many patients, unfortunately, would expire from systemic disease prior to any brain tumor recurrence, and for those patients, whole-brain radiotherapy would ultimately have no benefit. In addition, whole-brain radiotherapy is only marginally effective as a prophylactic against development of future brain metastasis, and would of course not result in improved outcome for those patients for whom the treatment would not actually succeed. These later recurrences can result from failure to control existing subclinical deposits a well as later seeding with tumor cells that were not present when radiotherapy was administered. Finally, salvage treatment with later radiosurgery, surgery, or whole-brain radiotherapy is available for those who have subsequent intracranial recurrences. Indeed, for individual patients to expire as a result of omitting whole-brain radiotherapy, presupposes not only a recurrence within their lifetime, but also the fact that whole-brain radiotherapy might have been able to prevent that recurrence and that the recurrence could not have been controlled by the later therapies.

Several randomized trials have examined whole-brain radiotherapy when added to focal therapy versus focal therapy alone, although these trials were often powered with brain control or neurological death as a primary endpoint without power to demonstrated equivalence in absolute survival with any robustness. Nevertheless, the results have been consistent in that no survival benefit has been suggested. Patchell (1) has reported the results of a trial that included patients with a resected single brain metastasis and Karnofsky performance status ≥70 who were randomized to therapy with or without postoperative adjuvant whole brain radiotherapy. Although the most commonly used palliative dose of radiotherapy in routine practice is 30–35 cGy over 2–3 weeks to be respectful of patients' time, a higher dose of radiation was utilized in this trial—50.4 Gy at 1.8 Gy per day over 5 weeks—to maximize the chances of demonstrating a benefit in tumor control. In addition, lower fraction sizes such as 1.8 cGy per day appeared to reduce toxicity compared with higher daily doses.

The results of this trial are summarized in Table 6.1. Although there was a meaningful benefit in local control at the operative site and reduced later brain metastasis elsewhere in the brain, there was no survival benefit or better functional independence with whole-brain radiotherapy. The authors concluded that whole-brain radiotherapy should be standard even after resection of a single brain metastasis because there was a decreased chance of subjectively assessed neurological death and because there was very high local and distant

TABLE 6.1  Benefit to Postoperative Whole-Brain Radiotherapy—Randomized, Patchell et al. (1)

|  | SURGERY ALONE | SURGERY/RT (5,040 RADS) |
| --- | --- | --- |
| Survival | 43 weeks | 48 weeks |
| Brain recurrence | 70% | 18% |
| Original site | 46% | 10% |
| Other sites | 37% | 14% |
| Neurologic death | 44% | 14% |

brain combined recurrence rate after surgery alone, which was substantially reduced by the addition of WBRT. It must be emphasized that this trial was powered to detect a reduction in brain recurrence, with survival analysis as a secondary endpoint. Thus, this trial was not intended either to demonstrate or rule out a modest improvement in survival outcome.

A cautionary (2) editorial that accompanied the above article by Patchell, published in the *Journal of the American Medical Association*, present the view that the data presented might not be sufficient to dictate postoperative radiotherapy as a clear-cut standard of care for all applicable patients after surgical resection:

> But it is uncertain whether all patients should receive postoperative radiation, as they suggest, when median survival time and length of functional independence are not enhanced by early treatment. The authors argue that "neurologic death . . . is most difficult for patients and their families. . . . " While acknowledging their point of view, it is important to note that nonneurologic symptoms including nausea, breathlessness, and pain can also be difficult to endure, witness, and manage. Moreover, had fatigue, alopecia, eustachian tube dysfunction, memory loss, and other adverse effects of radiation been considered, and had quality of life been measured, it might be less clear that early whole-brain radiation is the "right" choice for all patients whose single brain metastasis has been fully resected. Individualized treatment decisions, guided by the results of important trials like this one, always will have an important place in clinical medicine.

An ongoing randomized trial of the European Organization for Research and Therapy of Cancer (EORTC) is even now initiating a study of patients to reevaluate the role of standard whole-brain radiotherapy after resection of brain metastasis in comparison with observation. Others (3) are investigating the role of radiosurgery as focal postoperative therapy to the resection cavity alone, to treat the highest risk area postoperatively while avoiding prophylactic therapy of uninvolved brain. Large data sets of this new approach are not yet available to provide guidance.

As discussed elsewhere in this text, focal radiosurgery is a commonly used alternative to surgical resection that may be appropriate treatment for gross lesions for a greater percentage of patients in that deeper lesions and multiple sites can be treated even in the presence of other comorbidities, The potential for a survival benefit from adjuvant whole brain radiotherapy might be even lower in these nonoperative patients, as radiosurgery alone appears to result in a substantially lower baseline risk of actual tumor bed recurrence compared with conventional surgery alone, which may diminish the need for adjuvant therapies. Although counterintuitive, this is perhaps the result of the significant radiation dose deposited into the immediately adjacent at-risk brain. On the other hand, surgical candidates might be in better overall condition with more limited disease and may therefore have a higher chance of benefiting from better control of tumor in the brain.

Aoyama (4) has reported the results of a randomized trial conducted in Japan (JROSG99-1) for patients with 1–4 metastasis and KPS ≥70 who were treated by radiosurgery with or without whole-brain radiotherapy. These results are summarized in Table 6.2 and are generally similar to the results reported by Patchell after surgical resection. As expected, these data demonstrate a higher brain control rate but have not demonstrated benefits to survival, neurological death, or maintenance of good performance status. Whole-brain radiotherapy did not improve survival, performance status, or neurologic survival, and there was no evidence of survival benefit. Brain tumor recur-

TABLE 6.2  Results of JROSG99-1—Randomized, Aoyoma et al. (4)

|  | RS ALONE | RS AND WBRT |
|---|---|---|
| 1 year survival | 28% | 39% (p=NS) |
| Neurologic death | 15% | 10% (p=NS) |
| 1 year KPS ≥70 | 25% | 37% (P=NS) |
| 1 year new mets | 51% | 28% (P=.003) |
| 1 year local failure | 30% | 12% (p=.019) |
|  | WBRT + SRS | SRS |
| 1 year intracranial recurrence | 46.8% | 76.4% |
| 1 year new metastases | 41.5% | 63.7% |
| 1 year local control | 88.7% | 72.5% |
| Overall survival | 38.5% | 28.4% |
| Median survival | 7.5 months | 8.0 months |
| Neurologic death | 22.8% | 19.3% |
| Neurologic preservation | 72.1% | 70.3% |

rence is more frequent when whole brain radiotherapy is omitted, and the authors emphasize that it should therefore only be omitted when close follow-up of the patient is possible. Of note, distant brain tumor recurrence was more frequent after whole-brain treatment than in Patchell's results and may relate to the inclusion of patients with multiple metastasis at baseline, use of a different whole brain radiotherapy schedule, and other unknown selection factors.

Chougule (5) has reported in abstract form a modestly powered 96 patient three arm randomized trial that included whole-brain radiotherapy, radiosurgery alone, and whole-brain radiotherapy in conjunctions with radiosurgery for patients with 1–3 lesions. Radiosurgery was 20 Gy. Fifty-one patients had resection of a large symptomatic lesion, in which case the tumor bed was treated with radiosurgery. Median survival was 7, 5, and 9 months for the radiosurgery, radiosurgery + WBRT and WBRT arms, respectively, and local control of the treated lesions was 87 percent, 91 percent, and 62 percent, respectively, confirming a local benefit from radiosurgery However, the occurrence of new brain lesions was lower (43 percent, 19 percent, and 23 percent, respectively) in the two arms receiving WBRT. These data, although the trial is underpowered, suggest brain control but not survival benefit from the addition of whole-brain radiotherapy and are consistent with the results of JROSG99-1 (described above) as well as with the trial reported by Patchell.

Two other international randomized trials are currently assembling a patient cohort to test the benefit of whole brain radiotherapy after radiosurgey. EORTC 22952 is enrolling patients with 1–3 metastasis and WHO is conducting performance status on patients with 0–2 metastasis who have previously had resection of a brain metastasis and/or are planning to get radiosurgery. Patients will be randomized to receive or not receive whole-brain radiotherapy. A U.S. Intergroup trial, North Central Cancer Treatment Group (NCCTG) N0574, which will also be populated through the Eastern Cooperative Oncology Group (ECOG), the American College of Surgeons Oncology Group (ACOSOG), and the Cancer Trials Support Unit (CTSU) is being initiated, but enrollment of patients for this trial has been slow. In this trial patients with 1–3 metastasis will be randomized to radiosurgery with or without whole-brain radiotherapy. Both trials will address not only survival and brain recurrence, but also quality of life and neurocognitive endpoints. These trials, in combination with mature results from JROSG99-1, should provide valuable quantitative data about the important oncologic and quality of life endpoints that patients and physicians should weigh when picking a treatment option.

Several large retrospective analyses provide additional supporting evidence that there is unlikely to be a significant survival decrement resulting from omission of WBRT, although this has not been a universal finding and these series are certainly subject to selection biases. Gerosa (6) reported survival outcome for 804 patients with KPS ≥60 treated for 1,307 lesions, and survival outcome was superior to that which would have been expected from whole-brain radiotherapy without radiosurgery, likely reflecting a positive selection bias but also suggesting that survival is not shortened by omission of whole-brain radiotherapy. Median survival was 14 months and actuarial 1 year local progression free survival at the treated lesion site was 93 percent. In the most extensive review of this kind, Sneed (7) has reported retrospectively acquired data from multiple institutions describing survival outcome for patients treated with and without radiosurgery. Forty percent of patients had more than one lesion. The results are summarized in Table 6.3, which shows no evidence of a survival benefit even when patients are grouped according to the Radiation Therapy Oncology Group (RTOG) recursive partitioning analysis (RPA) classification. In a separate retrospective analysis, Sneed (8) reported that although brain recurrence was more common without whole-brain radiation, allowing for one episode of salvage treatment, the odds of brain control at any point in time appeared similar. Finally, in this large data set, Sneed found no survival benefit from whole-brain radiotherapy, even for patients with large numbers of metastases, suggesting that omitting whole-brain radiotherapy is an appropriate option for selected and motivated patients, even with extensive numbers of lesions.

Kondziolka (9) reviewed long-term survivors of gamma knife therapy (4 or more years) and compared these patients with short-term survivors to test the hypothesis that long-term survival would be less likely without whole-brain

TABLE 6.3 Retrospective Comparison, Sneed et al. (7)

|                    | RADIOSURG | WBRT + RADIOSURG |
|--------------------|-----------|------------------|
| Number             | 268       | 301              |
| Median surv        | 8.2 m     | 8.6 m            |
| 1 year surv        | 38%       | 35%              |
| Median surv Class I | 14 m     | 15 m             |
| Class II           | 8 m       | 7 m              |
| Class III          | 5 m       | 5 m              |
| Further Tx         | 37%       | 7%               |

radiotherapy. There was no difference in these populations related to the use of whole-brain radiotherapy, and many patients required several episodes of radiosurgery over this period of time. Long-term survival was associated with better performance status, fewer brain metastases, and less extracranial disease when compared with outcomes of whole-brain radiotherapy.

In another interesting retrospective report, Varlotto (10) reported results for patients who survived 1 or more year after stereotactic radiosurgery (SRS) at the University of Pittsburgh to evaluate whether WBRT may contribute to actual long-term distant brain control or whether the benefit might be transient and not significantly relevant to long-term outcome. Distant brain control (Table 6.4) was only modestly improved, and recurrence was common with or without WBRT. This analysis, although retrospective, suggests that WBRT may be only marginally beneficial in controlling tumor in the brain in the long run. This may be a result not only of failure to control existing disease but also the possibility that many brain failures may result from later reseeding that cannot be addressed by immediate WBRT. The 1, 3, and 5 year failure rates were 26 percent, 75 percent, and 75 percent in 40 patients treated with SRS alone versus 21 percent, 49 percent, and 62 percent in 69 patients treated with WBRT along with SRS.

Randomized data, prospective data, and retrospective data, therefore, are all consistent in suggesting an absence of survival benefit with whole-brain radiotherapy, although the limited size of the randomized trials has not justified definitive conclusions that eliminate all controversy surrounding this issue. Brain tumor recurrence is common, and decisions are often based on the competing risk of tumor recurrence and treatment-related toxicity.

## Toxicity: A Reason to Avoid Whole-Brain Radiotherapy

WBRT has been associated with acute and late toxicities that have motivated physicians and patients to avoid utilizing this therapy if possible. Acute effects

TABLE 6.4 Distant Brain Failure in Long-Term Survivors. Retrospective, Varlotto et al. (10)

| >1 YEAR SURVIVORS | 1 YEAR FAILURE | 3 YEAR FAILURE | 5 YEAR FAILURE |
| --- | --- | --- | --- |
| Gamma Knife (40) | 26 ± 7% | 75 ± 10% | 75 ± 9% |
| With WBRT (69) | 21 ± 5% | 49 ± 9% | 62 ± 13% |

of treatment include substantial fatigue, hair loss, skin effects, otitis media, significant fatigue, and the need for corticosteroids. The symptoms frequently persist for several months and may be of substantial importance to the bulk of patients who will survive less than a year, most often dying from progressive systemic cancer rather than brain failure. These effects are not well studied but are commonly observed in clinical practice. In a survey study (11) of subjective complaints in patients treated with whole-brain radiotherapy along with radiosurgery, 69 percent complained of excess fatigue, 60 percent reported decreased short-term memory, 29 percent reported decreased long-term memory, 44 percent complained about depression, and 13 percent expressed concern that their hair had not grown back. These complaints were uncommon in a comparison group treated with radiosurgery alone, and this may be of critical importance to many patients whose illness will likely result in relatively near-term death.

Late neurocognitive sequelae have been reported as well and are of great concern for those destined to be long-term survivors. DeAngelis, et al. (12) reported on 12 patients treated with WBRT at a dose of 25–39 Gy in 3 to 6 Gy fractions. These patients were all found to have dementia, ataxia, and incontinence at a median of 14 months after treatment. Indeed, smaller fraction sizes are used in modern practice, and the actual incidence of radiation-induced fulminant dementia is likely much lower. Studies using these regimens in conjunction with neurocognitive follow-up have suggested general stability in neurocognitive function for most patients in the short to medium term after whole-brain radiotherapy in the absence of tumor recurrence.

Imaging studies confirm a structural effect of radiation even at modest doses typically used for palliative whole-brain radiotherapy. In a study of 90 patients (13), the mean atrophy index was 1.08 + 0.18, 1.21 + 0.33 at 3 months and 1.28 + 0.4, 1.37 + .44, and 1.43 + 0.52 at 3, 6, 12, and 18 months after radiotherapy (RT). At 6 and 12 months, 30 percent and 47 percent had an atrophy index greater than 1.3. Mini-mental state exam declined only in a small percentage of patients with this follow-up, but this is an insensitive test and evaluation including true neurocognitive testing is essential to detect the more subtle but very meaningful dysfunction that is likely to occur with follow-up over this limited period. Other studies have demonstrated a measurable change on MRI spectroscopy and T2 MRI as a long-term visible representation of the effects of radiation. Recently, Diffusion Tensor MRI (14) has demonstrated the ability to detect early radiation related structural changes even as early as one month posttherapy.

# A Toxicity of Omitting Whole-Brain Radiotherapy: Risk of Symptomatic Brain Tumor Recurrence

The risk of developing new lesions in the brain is higher when whole-brain radiotherapy is not utilized, and a preventable recurrence could potentially cause neurological symptoms or injury. This could be considered a potential "toxicity" of omitting whole-brain radiotherapy. This possibility must be weighed against the actual toxicity of whole-brain therapy and has not been rigorously studied.

Regine (15) reported that, of 36 patients treated with radiosurgery alone for brain metastasis, 47 percent (17 patients) had a recurrence in the brain, and 71 percent (ten or 28 percent of originally treated patients) had neurological symptoms at recurrence. The ultimate impact of this is unknown, as only some of these recurrences would likely have been prevented by whole-brain radiotherapy and some symptomatic recurrences undoubtedly responded favorably to steroids and salvage treatment. Similarly, Lauterbach (16) reported that 38 percent of patients had recurrence diagnosed by symptoms rather than by routine MRI. Other series involving radiosurgery alone have generally not reported the symptomatic impact of recurrence.

Importantly, tumor progression, as well as treatment toxicity, may also be an important cause of neurocognitive decline, not just focal deficits. Myers (17) reported the results of a large data set of patients prospectively evaluated with neurocognitive testing after whole-brain radiation and found that decline was most associated with tumor progression. There was no comparison group treated with focal radiotherapy alone, and many likely had disease that was too extensive, making it unclear whether a group treated with focal radiotherapy would have fared better overall. But this data does highlight the issue of the damage that can be caused by recurrence. The Japanese randomized trial reported by Aoyama (18) included follow-up evaluation using the insensitive mini-mental state test, and it was not clear that outcome differed with or without whole-brain treatment. Recently reported short-term results of an RTOG trial (19) that included neurocognitive testing demonstrated that a majority of patients showed improvement one month after whole-brain radiotherapy, possibly as a result of beneficial effects on tumor. Longer-term data, however, is clearly needed.

The possibility that recurrence may be an avoidable cause of functional decline for some patients is certainly a reason for caution and for fully involving the patient in the decision process. This risk should generally be a part of discussions with any patient considering WBRT. Very timely MRI follow-up for patients in otherwise good condition might be appropriate to detect asymptomatic recurrence whether or not radiosurgery is utilized. The ongoing randomized trials, which address various quality of life endpoints, should ultimately provide important data beyond that which is currently available to inform this decision-making process.

## Criteria for Offering the Choice of Focal Therapy Alone

The data do not provide clear guidelines for patient selection for this option. The possibility of higher risk of later lesions requiring treatment suggests it should be offered to motivated patients who will comply with rigorous follow-up, although even after whole-brain radiation there remains a substantial risk of new lesions that necessitates close follow-up except in those patients who are in a terminal condition from systemic tumor. The data described above also suggests that if the number of metastases is greater than 3 or 4, especially if they are large or there is active systemic disease, the rate of later distant brain failure may be high enough that whole-brain radiotherapy should be strongly considered. Similar considerations likely apply to patients who have had surgical resection.

Local therapy should be offered to well-selected patients who are likely to benefit from this costly and more aggressive approach. Randomized trials have shown a benefit when resection and/or radiosurgery is added to whole-brain radiotherapy for 1–3 metastases in patients with good performance status. These patients are generally treated with radiosurgery, and the patient care issue is whether to add whole-brain radiotherapy rather than substitute radiosurgery for less costly whole-brain treatment. Indeed, the available data suggests that omission of whole-brain radiotherapy can be appropriately discussed with most patients in that category.

Patients with substantially more than 3 lesions or bulky lesions may be more likely to have near-term brain tumor recurrence, but the omission of whole-brain radiotherapy may be considered after careful consideration and discussion of the risks of recurrence and the need for rigorous follow-up. As need for additional treatment in the near and medium term is high and may be reduced by whole-brain radiotherapy, the countervailing benefits should be explicitly considered for each patient's individual circumstances. Potential additional factors to consider are that (1) radiosurgery does not generally require a length delay until institution of systemic therapy, and this may be important in the care of many patients; (2) this treatment causes less disruption to normal activity such as work or vacation plans; (3) there are fewer short-term quality of life effects and a lower time commitment for those who may have only limited survival expectations; and (4) there is a potentially improved neurocognitive outcome for long-term survivors. For patients with poor performance status and/or predicted survival less than 3 months, the costs of the therapy may be harder to justify, but the short time commitment involved and minimal side effects may be an important advantage under carefully selected circumstances.

Local therapy would most ideally be offered as a choice for patients if there is a relative likelihood for long interval before need for future treatment, although reduced treatment-related toxicity might still reasonably motivate patients to attempt to avoid whole-brain radiotherapy and even prefer repeated applications of radiosurgery. Relevant data is reviewed below.

In the randomized trial of Aoyama, the following factors were associated with increased risk of distant brain failure including 2 or more metastases (hazard rate 1.69), presence of extracranial metastasis (hazard rate 2.06), and KPS <90 (hazard rate 2.14). Sawrie (20) reported similar predictive factors for distant brain failure after focal therapy alone in a retrospective analysis, reasoning that if a group could be identified with a very high risk, whole-brain therapy might be most appropriate. Interestingly, a favorable group consisting of those with fewer than 4 metastases, no existing extracranial disease, and non-melanoma histology had a median time to distant brain failure of 89 weeks versus 33 weeks for those with 1 or more of these characteristics. The 1-year probability of freedom from distant brain failure was 46 percent for three or fewer metastases, whereas it was 0 percent for 4 or more, 27 percent for melanoma versus 40 percent for other histologies, and 68 percent versus 30 percent for the presence or absence of extracranial disease. In multivariate analyses, the number of metastases and extracranial disease were significant. Although it may still be a reasonable treatment choice for those with higher risk of distant brain tumor recurrence, the likely need for repeated treatments and risk of symptomatic new lesions should be considered within the context of each patient's goals and medical situation.

The approach may be suitable for certain patients with 4 or more lesions, but patients choosing this option must be willing to accept the high likelihood of need for further therapy. In an analysis by Lorenzoni (21), the presence of more than three lesions and up to nine lesions was not prognostic for survival after radiosurgery alone. Yan (22) reported that when radiosurgery was utilized with or without whole-brain radiotherapy, survival was similar for those with 1, 2, 3, 4–5, 6–7, and >8 lesions. Total target volume, age <65, KPS ≥70, and absence of extracranial disease were prognostic for better survival outcome. Amendola (23) reported radiosurgery alone results for patients with 10 or more metastases, with a reasonable survival outcome for those with KPS ≥70 and especially with small volume disease less than 30 cm³.

The authors have analyzed outcome for 98 patients treated (24) with radiosurgery for brain metastasis. One year and median survivals for patients with three or fewer lesions was 38 percent and 8.4 months versus 32 percent (n=66) and 6.7 months for those with more than four lesions (n=32). Median survivals were 8.4 and 6.7 months, respectively (p=NS). Survival did not appear to be affected by the use of prior whole-brain radiotherapy. Generally, patients with four or more lesions treated with radiosurgery alone or with whole-brain radiotherapy represent a highly selected group who may have small volume disease despite the number of lesions, a good performance status, and may have even had some of the lesions identified only on thin-cut MRI performed on the day of the procedure after the frame was placed. The data justifying this approach is retrospective, and it is likely these represent selected groups of patients who had good performance status and smaller lesions.

Indeed, the more likely determinant of outcome after SRS is a change in overall tumor volume. Bhatnagar (25), in a retrospective study of patients who received SRS for >=4 metastases, found that total tumor volume, and not the number of brain metastases, was predictive of overall survival. A similar report by Kim (26) also demonstrated a significant correlation of survival with total intracranial tumor volume (Table 6.5), but not with the use of WBRT or the number of metastases. Yan et al. (22) also reported total tumor volume, rather

TABLE 6.5 Survival is Related to Total Volume of Brain Metastasis, Kim et al. (26).

| VOLUME (CC) | SURVIVAL (MONTHS) |
| --- | --- |
| <1 | 10.2 |
| 1–4.9 | 8.5 |
| 5–14.9 | 5.3 |
| >15 | 3.6 |

than absolute number of metastases, as prognostic. Yu et al. (27) found intracranial tumor volume and presence of extracranial disease to be prognostic in patients treated for metastatic melanoma. Thus, intracranial tumor volume may prove to be another appropriate tool to assess patients' eligibility for SRS. There is currently no established cut-off value for tumor volume in patient selection for SRS alone, and this issue requires further study.

Given this limited data, it is not possible to develop clear guidelines for selection. The treatment selection should be highly individualized, and may be most dependent on meaningful discussion of the patients' own views of the trade-offs. Patients should be counseled on the toxicities of the therapeutic options, and the high likelihood of need for salvage treatment for repeated recurrences after focal therapy for 4 or more lesions or bulky lesions. For many patients, the clear demonstration for a reduction in the relative risk of developing a new brain metastasis justifies a decision for whole-brain radiotherapy. This decision may be motivated by a simple desire to reduce the risks of new brain lesions, the fear of symptomatic recurrence, or the desire to reduce the chances of needing future treatment. However, other patients may appropriately and knowingly choose an option that leads to a high risk of requiring more treatment in the future because of the absence of a proven survival benefit as well as because of the toxicities and burdens of treatment that may affect a significant portion of remaining survival time. For patients for whom surgical resection or radiosurgery is an appropriate option and in situations where all known intracranial disease has been treated, consideration of the alternative of omitting whole-brain radiotherapy is therefore reasonable and justified even as we await the results of randomized trials that will likely provide data that will better define the trade-offs involved in this decision and inform the choices that must be made by individual patients and physicians.

# References

1. Patchell RA, Tibbs PA, Regine WF, et al. Postoperative radiotherapy in the treatment of single metastases to the brain: A randomized trial. *JAMA* 1998;280:1485–1489.
2. Mintz AP, Cairncross JG. Treatment of a single brain metastasis: The role of radiation following surgical resection. *JAMA* 1998;280:1527–1529.
3. Do L, Pezner RD, Radeny E., et al. Resection followed by stereotactic radiosurgery to the resection cavity for 1–4 intracranial metastases. *Int J Radiat Oncol Biol Phys* 2007;69(3): S247–248.
4. Aoyama H, Shirato H, Tago M, et al. Stereotactic radiosurgery plus whole-brain radiation therapy versus stereotactic radiosurgery alone for treatment of brain metastases: A randomized controlled trial. *JAMA* 2006;295:2483–2491.

5. Chougule PB, Burton-Williams M, Saris S et al. Randomized treatment of brain metastasis with gamma knife radiosurgery, whole-brain radiotherapy or both. *Int J Radiat Oncol Biol Phys* 2000;48:114.

6. Gerosa M, Nicolato A, Foroni R, et al. Gamma knife radiosurgery for brain metastases: A primary therapeutic option. *J Neurosurg* 2002;97:515–524.

7. Sneed PK, Suh JH, Goetsch SJ, et al. A multi-institutional review of radiosurgery alone versus radiosurgery with whole brain radiotherapy as the initial management of brain metastases. *Int J Radiat Oncol Biol Phys* 2002;53:519–526.

8. Sneed PK, Lamborn KR, Forstner JM, et al. Radiosurgery for brain metastases: Is whole brain radiotherapy necessary? *Int J Radiat Oncol Biol Phys* 1999;43:549–558.

9. Kondziolka D, Martin JJ, Flickinger JC, et al. Long-term survivors after gamma knife radiosurgery for brain metastases. *Cancer* 2005;104:2784–2791.

10. Varlotto JM, Flickinger JC, Niranjan A, et al. The impact of whole-brain radiation therapy on the long-term control and morbidity of patients surviving more than one year after gamma knife radiosurgery for brain metastases. *Int J Radiat Oncol Biol Phys* 2005;62:1125–1132.

11. Kondziolka D, Niranjan A, Flickinger JC, et al. Radiosurgery with or without whole-brain radiotherapy for brain metastases: The patients' perspective regarding complications. *Am J Clin Oncol* 2005;28:173–179.

12. DeAngelis LM, Delattre JY, Posner JB. Radiation-induced dementia in patients cured of brain metastases. *Neurology* 1989;39:789–796.

13. Shibamoto Y, Baba FO, da K, et al. Incidence of brain atrophy and dementia after whole-brain radiotherapy in patients with brain metastases: A prospective study. *Int J Radiat Oncol Biol Phys* 2006;66:S86.

14. Nagesh V, Chenevert TL, Tsien CI, et al. Quantitative characterization of radiation dose dependent changes in normal appearing white matter of cerebral tumor patients using diffusion tensor imaging. *Int J Radiat Oncol Biol Phys* 2006;66:S4.

15. Regine WF, Huhn JL, Patchell RA, et al. Risk of symptomatic brain tumor recurrence and neurologic deficit after radiosurgery alone in patients with newly diagnosed brain metastases: Results and implications. *Int J Radiat Oncol Biol Phys* 2002;52:333–338.

16. Lutterbach J, Cyron D, Henne K, et al. Radiosurgery followed by planned observation in patients with one to three brain metastases. *Neurosurgery* 2003;52:1066–1073, discussion 1073–1074.

17. Meyers CA, Smith JA, Bezjak A, et al. Neurocognitive function and progression in patients with brain metastases treated with whole-brain radiation and motexafin gadolinium: Results of a randomized phase III trial. *J Clin Oncol* 2004;22:157–165.

18. Aoyama H, Tago M, Kato N, et al. Neurocognitive function of patients with brain metastasis who received either whole brain radiotherapy plus stereotactic radiosurgery or radiosurgery alone. *Int J Radiat Oncol Biol Phys* 2007;68:1388-1395.

19. Kwok Y, Won M, Regine WF, Mehta M, Schmitt F, Patchell RA, Watkins-Bruner D. Neurocognitive impact of whole brain radiation on patients with brain metastases: Secondary analysis of RTOG BR-0018. *Int J Radiat Oncol Biol Phys* 2007;69:S103.

20. Sawrie SM, Guthrie BL, Spencer SA, et al. Predictors of distant brain recurrence for patients with newly diagnosed brain metastases treated with stereotactic radiosurgery alone. *Int J Radiat Oncol Biol Phys* 2008;70:181–186.

21. Lorenzoni J, Devriendt D, Massager N, et al. Radiosurgery for treatment of brain metastases: Estimation of patient eligibility using three stratification systems. *Int J Radiat Oncol Biol Phys* 2004;60:218–224.

22. Yan ES, Sneed PK, McDermott MW, Kunwar S, Wara WM, Larson DA. Number of brain metastases is not an important prognostic factor for survival following radiosurgery for newly diagnosed nonmelanoma brain metastases. *Int J Radiat Oncol Biol Phys* 2003;57(2S)S131–132.

23. Amendola BE, Wolf A, Coy S, et al. Radiosurgery as palliation for brain metastases: A retrospective review of 72 patients harboring multiple lesions at presentation. *J Neurosurg* 2002;97:511–514.

24. Fox JL, Wharam M, Rigamonti D, et al. Can whole brain radiation be omitted in patients receiving radiosurgery for solitary or multiple brain metastases? *Int J Radiat Oncol Biol Phys* 2006;66:S251–S252.

25. Bhatnagar AK, Flickinger JC, Kondziolka D, et al. Stereotactic radiosurgery for four or more intracranial metastases. *Int J Radiat Oncol Biol Phys* 2006;64:898-903.

26. Kim EY, Macinas RJ, Willliams JM, et al. Tumor volume is a predictor for overall survival for patients with brain metastasis who undergo gamma knife stereotactic radiosurgery. *Int J Radiat Oncol Biol Phys* 2006;66:S86.

27. Yu C, Chen JC, Apuzzo ML, et al. Metastatic melanoma to the brain: Prognostic factors after gamma knife radiosurgery. *Int J Radiat Oncol Biol Phys* 2002;52:1277–1287.

# 7

# Chemotherapy for Brain Metastasis
## What We Know and What We Don't

Erin M. Dunbar

Brain metastases represent a heterogeneous group of systemic tumor histologies, which occur in an even more heterogeneous group of patients. Faced with the reality that the incidence of brain metastases continues to increase worldwide, the international medical community has met this challenge with enhanced dedication and new strategies. Historically, chemotherapy has served a minor role, often used predominantly for palliation and only after all surgery and radiation options were exhausted. Factors contributing to the minor role of chemotherapy in brain metastases include a lack of trials dedicated to brain metastases, a lack of agents demonstrating efficacy, and a lack of appreciation for the benefits of long-term brain control. However, thanks to the efforts of the patients, physicians, and researchers who have contributed to the information reviewed below, those factors are no longer lacking in the care of brain metastases.

The current standard options for patients able to receive aggressive therapy include a combination of surgery, radiation, and sometimes chemotherapy. Nonchemotherapy options are the focus of other chapters and will only be discussed in reference to their relationship to chemotherapy for brain metastases. Instead, the following chapter will review the factors related to the use of chemotherapy in brain metastases. It will review the evidence available for the incorporation of chemotherapy into the multidisciplinary management of brain metastases. It will emphasize the importance of collection and analysis of serial tissue and development of histology-specific clinical trials. Finally, it will highlight that careful balance must be maintained, including the balance between the outcomes of various treatment modalities, the balance between the focus on the brain and on the body, and a balance between the length and quality of life.

## Factors Determining Incidence

The incidence of brain metastases in the U.S. population is higher than ever. It is estimated that symptomatic brain metastases alone will develop in ~10 percent of adults with cancer during their lifetime (1,2). However, it is also estimated that at least 20 to 40 percent of adult cancer patients will develop asymptomatic brain metastases during their lifetime (3). When the total population of tumors occurring within the brain are evaluated, more than 50 percent are attributed to brain metastases. Collectively, these ratios translate into an excess of 200,000 cases reported per year in the United States (4). Brain metastases have different histologies, with the literature consistently reporting ~50 percent lung cancer, ~15 percent breast cancer, ~12 percent melanoma, <10 percent colorectal cancer, and <10 percent adenocarcinoma of unknown primary tumors. Of the histologies listed here, melanoma and breast are most likely to present as multiple lesions (5). Numerous factors contribute to the ever-increasing in incidence of brain metastases (1). The U.S. population itself, estimated in 2006 to be ~300 million, continues to increase annually. People in the United States are living longer, with current estimates of life expectancy for both men and women in the mid-eighties. These combined factors result in a population whose median age continues to rise, with the number of people aged 65 or older estimated in 2004 to be 12 percent or ~35.9 million people (6). Moreover, advances in health care unintentionally contribute to the growing number of brain metastases cases. Detection of brain metastases, both symptomatic and asymptomatic, has increased as a results of the technological improvement and more prevalent utilization of magnetic resonance imaging (MRI). At the same time, the percentage of adult patients with cancer who eventually develop brain metastases has grown as a result of improved local and systemic therapies, including chemotherapy. The impact of lengthened patient lives on the incidence of brain metastases is also attributable to the judicious application of multimodality therapies and the increased adherence of evidenced-based medicine. Also influencing the growing incidence of brain metastases is the cumulative effect of increasing awareness and advocacy by physicians, patients and caregivers, media, insurance companies, and medical systems.

# Factors Determining Response

Brian metastases represent several unique challenges that limit the responsiveness of chemotherapy, including the blood-brain barrier (BBB), tumor characteristics, inherent chemo sensitivity, and acquired chemoresistance.

## Blood-Brain Barrier

The blood-brain barrier is a physical, chemical, electric, and osmotic barrier, composed of intracerebral blood vessels, specialized endothelium, modified astrocytic podocytes, and adjacent brain parenchyma. Special features of this BBB include intercellular endothelial tight junctions, membrane-associated P-glycoproteins, and intracellular multidrug resistance proteins. Interstitial and intracranial pressure dynamics add to the challenge of manipulating the BBB. In the normal brain, the BBB limits the passage of large and hydrophilic drugs, including contrast dye and chemotherapy. However, there are certain natural and iatrogenic situations in which there is at least partial disruption of the BBB, therefore allowing substances to at least partially traverse the BBB. Examples include infection, inflammation, ischemia, trauma, radiation, and the presence of certain malignancies. Clinically, brain metastases are known for their reliable and homogeneous uptake of contrast enhancement on computed tomography (CT) and MRI, suggesting at least partial disruption of the BBB (7). Although metastases demonstrate the permeability of contrast dye into the tumor, the amount and extent of chemotherapy permeability is much less clear (8). Despite the challenges, there is increasing translational research evidence of at least a partial and transient permeability of the BBB. Direct sampling of the metastatic tumor after systemic chemotherapy exposure, via in vivo micro-dialysis catheters or intraoperative specimen collections, have demonstrated variable concentrations of drug within tumor. Additionally, direct comparisons of tumor from the original systemic primary site and the subsequent brain metastasis have revealed that P-glycoproteins have similar levels of expression in the metastatic tumor as that of the systemic primary tumor and that multidrug-resistance genes can be differentially activated, depending on previous drug exposure (9). Importantly, in addition to translational research evidence, there is also increasing clinical evidence of responsiveness of some tumors to chemotherapy. The ability to measure the clinical evidence of chemotherapy response is complicated by the use of corticosteroids and anti-angiogenic agents, both known to independently alter BBB permeability. Collectively, the increasing evidence of chemotherapy response in the treatment of brain metastases has intensified translational and clinical efforts to preferentially bypass and/or manipulate the BBB. One of the many areas of active investigation is the differential exploitation of radiation, anti-angiogenic agents, and nanotechnology for the penetration of chemotherapy across the BBB.

## Tumor Characteristics

Systemic tumor histologies have different inherent predilections for the brain. Histologies with some of the highest predilections to metastasize to the brain include melanoma, small cell lung cancer, and germ cell tumors. Although a comprehensive review of this topic is beyond the scope of this chapter, existing evidence for the inherent predilections observed include the presence of embryological, chemotropic, vascular, and cancer stem cell factors that facilitate the metastasis of the cells from the primary systemic tumor into the central nervous system (CNS). In addition, the cytologic infrastructure of metastatic cells (including their organelles, receptors, and channels) may affect their responsiveness to chemotherapy. Indirectly, the size of the metastases and the surrounding microenvironment (including ischemia, hypoxia, acidity, and pressure gradients) may affect their responsiveness to chemotherapy. Similarly, heterogeneity within the ultrastructure of the metastases itself may result in varied disruption of the BBB and varied clusters of mutations. Collectively, these tumor characteristics prevent chemotherapy from providing consistent and clinically meaningful responses (10).

## Chemosensitivity

There is increasing translational and clinical evidence that selecting a chemotherapy that has demonstrated chemosensitivity with the primary systemic tumor is very important in predicting chemotherapy response in brain metastases (9). Some systemic tumor histologies, such as germ cell tumors or certain lymphomas, are significantly more "inherently" chemosensitive. However, obtaining high-quality evidence regarding the chemosensitivity of brain metastases has been historically limited by certain factors. Existing studies, for example, have often pooled results from post hoc analyses of larger studies, often including patients with uncontrolled or unmeasured systemic disease.

In addition, existing studies have often pooled results from both new and recurrent disease settings, often including patients with uncontrolled or unmeasured numbers of previous therapies. Finally, existing studies have often pooled results from trials indiscriminately including all histologies, often insufficiently reporting histology-specific chemotherapy response, pertinent outcome measures, or even the status of brain disease at death. Moreover, the criteria used to determine chemosensitivity is too often limited to radiographic response alone, which is at best, incomplete, and at worst, inaccurate. However, these historical limitations are being actively addressed through improved translational modeling, improved analysis of human tissue, and improved clinical trial design.

## Chemoresistance

The etiology and contributions of a brain metastasis' inherent chemosensitivity versus its acquired chemoresistance are not fully understood. However, analysis of serial tumor specimens and clinical experience support that at least a portion of the cancer cells that have metastasized to the brain have already acquired resistance to many drugs, including those originally used treat the systemic disease. Several prospective clinical trials and retrospective analyses report that patients who have not previously been treated with chemotherapy will experience response rates at their brain metastases that are comparable to those seen at their systemic site (11). In contrast, patients who have already been treated with chemotherapy, will experience response rates at their brain metastases that are less impressive (12). There are many reasons for this difference in clinical experience. Patients initially presenting with widely metastatic disease, including the brain metastases, are likely biologically different from those developing meta-synchronous metastases to the brain at progression. In vivo and in vitro translational research evidence are beginning to unlock the etiology and contributions of this differential chemosensitivity, and clinical researchers are anxious to exploit them.

## Factors Determining Treatment Strategy

Currently, the standard treatment options for patients with brain metastases include symptom control, surgery, whole brain radiation therapy (WBRT), and stereotactic radiosurgery (SRS). Multiple factors help determine the ideal selection for an individual patient.

## Standard Treatment Options

For patients who desire treatment, and have controlled systemic disease, good prognostic factors, and one brain metastasis, the standard practice is maximally safe surgery followed by either WBRT or SRS. For those for whom surgery is not a safe option or the metastasis is in a surgically inaccessible location, SRS delivers equivalent results. The above strategy can be used in some patients with a limited number of metastases. WBRT is used, along with surgery or SRS, to prevent local and brain recurrence. Alternatively, in the setting of multiple brain metastases and palliation, WBRT can be used alone.

The median survival of those treated with only corticosteroids or only surgery is ~1 to 2 months or ~3 months, respectively (13). In comparison, prospective randomized trials demonstrate that the median survival with WBRT alone is ~4 to 6 months. Those treated with more than one modality, such as surgery followed by WBRT or surgery followed by SRS, have an enhanced survival by several weeks. There is definitive, albeit modest, improvement in the endpoints of local control, brain control, survival, and quality of life with these modalities. However, until definitive benefit can be demonstrated for chemotherapy with these endpoints, the use of chemotherapy will remain somewhat ancillary and palliative.

## Prognostic Factors

Careful analysis of large studies of patients with brain metastases has identified factors that predict an improved response and overall survival. These factors have been developed into validated prognostic criteria that can be used to tailor available therapies to the individual patient. One of the most frequently used, the recursive partitioning analysis (RPA) developed by the Radiation Therapy Oncology Group (RTOG), incorporates the factors of performance status, extent of extracranial disease, and age. This three class prognostic system has been validated with thousands pf patients (14–16). Class I (favorable prognosis) has Karnofsky performance score (KPS) >70, age <65, no extracranial metastases, a controlled primary tumor, and a median survival of 7.1 months. Class II (intermediate prognosis) has KPS >70, but with other unfavorable characteristics and a median survival of 4.2 months. Class III (poor prognosis) has a KPS <70 and a median survival of 2.3 months (15). Using these criteria, it is standard practice to offer RPA Class I and Class II patients multimodality therapy and RPA Class III patients either WBT alone or palliative care.

## Chemotherapy Agents

Thanks to a century of medical advancements, there has been an astonishing increase in the number of chemotherapeutic drug classes and resultant drug choices. Once faced with only minimal chemotherapeutic options, clinical researchers now must use preclinical models to select the subset of agents most likely to have clinical efficacy. Once faced with a more homogeneous population of patients considered candidates for chemotherapy, physicians now must acknowledge that both the patient population and clinical trials have changed. For instance, patents increasingly present with asymptomatic brain metastases, with the brain the only site of active disease. Likewise, patients tend to be in better overall health and better tolerate chemotherapy with the help of modern supportive care. Finally, clinical trials tend to be better equipped to answer chemotherapy-related preclinical and clinical questions.

## Outcomes

There has been a shift in the desired outcome measurements for therapies administered for brain metastases, including chemotherapy. Although the gold standard remains overall survival (OS), other endpoints, including clinical and/or radiographic response rate (RR), time to progression (TTP), and disease-free survival (DFS), have become more frequently used surrogates. In addition, neurologic status, overall performance (functional) status (PS), neurocognitive performance, quality of life (QOL), and healthcare utilization are becoming increasingly important endpoints. The latter is, at least in part, due to the collective advocacy of patients, their caregivers, the media, and the financial entities within health care. One illustration of many includes the previously held firm belief that incidentally found brain metastases were asymptomatic. However, recent research has eloquently shown that 65 percent of patients eventually diagnosed with brain metastases demonstrated cognitive impairment (usually in multiple domains) on detailed neurologic testing, even prior to their diagnoses (17). Determining where the latter outcome measurements will rank amongst the traditional endpoints will become a little clearer when the results of several multicenter phase II/III trials using them become available in the near future.

## Treatment Strategies Incorporating Chemotherapy

As in systemic malignancies, chemotherapy used for brain metastases can be combined in a variety of ways, either at diagnosis or at recurrence, either with other treatment modalities or alone, either with the goal of disease control or palliation.

### Concurrent Chemotherapy with Whole-Brain Radiation (WBRT)

Over the years, multiple chemotherapy agents have been administered with WBRT. Treatment has been administered in a concurrent, neo-adjuvant or adjuvant setting, either at new diagnosis or at recurrence. Some of the most common agents used in combination with radiation include nitrosureas, tenopiside, tegafur, the platinums, temozolomide, and a number of newer agents. Of the common agents listed here, temozolomide is of particular interest. Preclinically, this agent that has demonstrated radiosensitizing properties and has also demonstrated pronounced benefits both in tumors with certain histologies and tumors with a methylated MGMT (O(6)-methylguanine-DNA-methyltransferase) DNA repair enzyme (a.k.a. "silenced" or ineffective DNA repair enzyme). Further outlined in the individual histology sections below, the combination of temozolomide and WBRT has demonstrated improved radiographic responses, decreased neurologic toxicity, and improved quality of life. The following clinical trials with temozolomide illustrate the achievable impact of concurrent WBRT and chemotherapy. In a phase II trial, 52 patients with new brain metastases were randomly administered temozolomide ($75mg/m^2/day$) concurrently with standard WBRT (30 Gy) versus WBRT alone. The objective response rate was 96 percent (38 percent complete response and 58 percent partial response) for the combined versus 67 percent objective response (33 percent complete response and 33 percent partial response) for the WBRT alone (p = 0.017). In addition, fewer patients required corticosteroid therapy two months after treatment (67 percent versus 91 percent) (18). In another phase II trial, 82 patients with brain metastases were randomly administered WBT alone versus WBRT with concurrent temozolomide $75mg/m^2/day$, followed by 2 months of adjuvant temozolomide ($200mg/m^2/day$) on days 1–5 out of a 28-day month. In addition to the absence of any additional neurologic toxicity, the results of the concurrent arm supported improved brain control. Progression free survival (PFS) at 90 days was 54 percent for WBRT versus 72 percent for WBRT and temozolomide (p = 0.03), and death from brain metastases was higher in the WBRT alone arm (69 percent versus 41 percent) (p = 0.03) (19). A third phase II trial of 59 patients with brain metastases were all administered concurrent WBRT (30 Gy) and temozolomide ($75mg/m^2$/day), then followed by up to 6 months of temozolomide ($150mg/m^2$/day) on days 1–5 of a 28-day month. There were 5 patients with a complete response, 21 with a partial response, and 18 with stable disease. The overall response rate was 45 percent, the median time to progression was 9 months, and the median overall survival was 13 months. Using the FACT-G, there was a significant improvement in quality of life (p <0.0001) (20). Numerous exciting trials with concurrent temozolomide and WBRT are ongoing, including several evaluating the relationship between clinical response and MGMT-methylation status of the tumor. Unfortunately, other chemotherapy agents administered with WBRT for brain metastases have not demonstrated significant improvements in response rates, survival, quality of life, or performance status, when compared in trials to WBRT alone. This pertains to chemotherapy agents administered in the concurrent, adjuvant and neo-adjuvant settings with WBRT, and includes carboplatin, 5-fluorouracil, chloronitrosoureas, cisplatin, vinorelbine (21–23).

The successful combination of small molecule inhibitors and radiation in other tumors, including head and neck squamous cell carcinoma, has led to similar evaluations in brain metastases. One example includes the ongoing phase II trial RTOG 0320, which involves erlotinib, a small molecular inhibitor of the epidermal growth factor receptor's (EGFR) intracellular tyrosine kinase (TK) domain. This trial compares WBRT and SRS alone (arm 1) versus with TMZ (arm 2) or erlotinib (arm 3) in patients with 1–3 brain metastases from non-small cell lung cancer (NSCLC). Results from this and similar trials are eagerly anticipated.

Given the increasing role of stereotactic radiosurgery (SRS) in the management of brain metastases, it is worth noting that numerous trials underway are evaluating combinations of chemotherapy and SRS.

## Chemotherapy Alone

The role of chemotherapy, as a monotherapy, is yet to be fully defined. Settings for the use of chemotherapy include both new diagnosis and recurrence. Goals of therapy include control of the tumor, palliation of symptoms, or a combination. Historic success with chemotherapy has been variable, partly due to an evolving understanding of drug delivery, effective agents, and clinical trial design. The literature addresses a limited number of trials dedicated to the evaluation of brain metastases. Only a subset of these trials have been adequately designed or powered to answer either clinical histology-specific or preclinical translational questions. Despite these limitations, the collective review of these historical trials reveals the following important trends.

In general, the chemosensitivity of the primary systemic tumor to a given chemotherapy agent remains a very important predictor of chemosensitivity in the subsequent brain metastases. Additionally, the clinical response of chemotherapy in the treatment-naïve patient is typically better than the response in patients who have already received one or more treatments. Moreover, the historical limitations of chemotherapy for brain metastases have inspired current investigators to incorporate new strategies, including innovative screening profiles, delivery systems, and clinical trial design. As discussed in the histology-specific sections below, temozolomide is one of the most researched chemotherapy agents for use as a monotherapy, given its oral absorption, excellent CNS penetration, and distinction from other chemotherapy agents requiring activation (24). Its role in the treatment of brain metastases is still evolving, and there have been a few recent phase II and III trials evaluating its use in this patient population. Another chemotherapy evaluated as a monotherapy in brain metastases is methotrexate, and agent with excellent CNS penetration when administered systemically at sufficient doses. This is illustrated in a phase II trial of 31 patients with brain metastases who were administered methotrexate ($3.5gm/m^2$ once per cycle). After a median of 4 cycles, 28 percent of these patients achieved an objective radiographic response, 28 percent achieved stable disease, and 44 percent progressed. The median overall survival (n = 32) was 19.9 weeks (25). A variety of other chemotherapy agents have only been described in case reports or case series as potential monotherapy for brain metastases. Given the recent tremendous increase in chemotherapy classes and individual drugs, the role of chemotherapy as a monotherapy remains completely undefined.

Of particular note is the need to balance the potential benefits of extended, increased or concurrent dosing strategies with chemotherapy with the potential complications of immunosuppression, such as CD4+ lymphopenia or neutropenia, anemia, or organ-toxicity that result from systemic agents (26).

## Radiosensitizing Agents

Optimizing the effects of radiation on the tumor, with little to no effect on the remaining brain, remains of great interest to researchers and clinicians.

Decades of preclinical research have revealed radiosensitizing properties of many of these agents with radiation, in both in vitro tests and in vivo animal models. Some of these agents are traditional chemotherapies, while others include oxidation-reduction agents, small molecule inhibitors, and additional agents. Despite their preclinical radiosensitizing properties, none of these agents has yet resulted in clinically meaningful improvements for brain metastases. Even more disappointing are consistent reports of the associated increased toxicity and intolerability. Examples of these agents include supplemental oxygen, metronidazole, misonidazole, metoxafin gadolinium (MGd), efaproxiral (SR13), bromodeoxyuridine (BrdUrd), lonidamine, platinums, temozolomide, and others (27–31). In summary, with the exception of temozolomide and MGd, these agents have not demonstrated a statistically significant improved rate of tumor control, tolerance, quality of life, or survival (32). The latter, metoxafin gadolinium (MGd), a metalloporphyrin redox modulator with preferential action on tumor cells, is inspiring renewed interest in radiosensitizing agents with several recent phase III demonstrating a delayed neurologic decline in patients with non-small cell lung cancer (NSCLC) brain metastases (33). In the first of two recent phase III trials, over 400 patients with brain metastases of various histologies were administered WBRT (30Gy) with or without MGd (5 mg/kg). Results hinted at an improvement in overall neurologic function in the first group, with 63 percent of NSCLC patients demonstrating improvement in memory and executive function (34,35). These encouraging results helped to launch the second phase III trial of similar study design, which focused exclusively on over 550 NSCLC patients (36). Using validated measurement criteria and blinded centralized review, researchers found that there was a trend to increased time to neurologic progression, the primary endpoint in the study, in patients receiving MGd (15.4 with combination versus 10 months with RT alone). Survival was similar in both arms (~5 months). It is important no note that only patients who initiated WBRT within 3 weeks demonstrated improvement. The ability of MGd to improve neurologic functioning, quality of life, and potentially even overall outcomes, are being evaluated in numerous ongoing studies (37). Other chemotherapies, including temozolomide, 5-FU, platinums, and others have also demonstrated radiosensitizing properties with radiation. If applicable to the treatment of brain metastases, they are discussed below.

## Chemotherapy with BBB Manipulation

Reliable delivery of chemotherapy into brain tumors, whether primary or metastatic, has led many scientists to pursue ways of circumventing the multi-faceted BBB. Techniques have included delivering higher concentration of chemotherapy through BBB vessels, as well as disrupting the integrity of BBB vessels. This is illustrated by the administration of chemotherapy into the carotid artery, either with or without the use of osmotic blood brain barrier disruption agents, such as mannitol. To date, trials using this strategy (largely small case series, in both primary and metastatic brain tumors), have resulted in relatively modest efficacy and at the expense of moderate toxicities (38,39). Despite the somewhat disappointing historical results, international interest in BBB disruption is increasing as agents such as monoclonal antibodies, whose large size and properties limit BBB permeability, are becoming standard therapy in several systemic malignancies (40).

## Chemotherapy for Micrometastases

The goal of preventing the recurrence of brain metastases is increasingly focused on the treatment of micrometastases, felt to be insidiously present at the time of diagnosis. Until recently, the only modality demonstrating efficacy was prophylactic cranial irradiation (PCI). PCI has been standard practice for small cell lung cancer (SCLC) patients, with either limited-stage disease or good-performance extensive stage disease, who experienced a good systemic response to chemotherapy. Illustrating this is a recent phase II trial of patients with extensive stage SCLC who responded to chemotherapy, a trial which randomized patients to either PCI or no PCI. The patients administered PCI had a lower risk of subsequent symptomatic brain metastases (hazard ratio, 0.27; 95 percent confidence interval [CI], 0.16 to 0.44; p <0.001), with an increase in median disease-free survival of 14.7 weeks (PCI) versus 12.0 weeks (no PCI), and a median overall survival of 6.7 months (PCI) versus 5.4 months (no PCI). Researchers reported that, although PCI resulted in measurable side effects to this patient population, there was no clinically significant effect on the global health status of this population (41). So, although PCI has been shown to reduce the occurrence of subsequent SCLC brain metastases, many related issues require further evaluation. These include the optimal dose and timing of PCI, the measurement and management of long-term effects of PCI, the role of PCI in extensive-stage SCLC, and the role of PCI in other systemic malignancies with high predilection for brain metastases (42). Concern that PCI and other forms of radiation cause delayed neurocognitive compromise has fueled the pursuit on nonradiation strategies to treat micrometastases. Chemotherapy agents with excellent CNS penetration, including temozolomide, lapatinib, and many others, are currently under investigation.

## Considerations for Certain Histologies

The optimal treatment of brain metastases is increasingly based on an in-depth understanding of its histology of origin. Ideally, this requires not only a basic confirmation of the histology of the metastasis, but also a precise analysis of its individual molecular and genetic features. Only then can chemotherapies be tailored to exploit a unique profile. Similarly, the heterogeneity of tumor characteristics—chemosensitivity, chemoresistance, and the BBB—makes comparative analysis of serial biopsies from a given patient extremely valuable.

The efficacy of chemotherapy in select histologies, including lung cancer, breast cancer, and melanoma, will be discussed below. These histologies were partly chosen for their frequency for metastasizing to the brain and were partly chosen for their relatively good response to chemotherapy. Some histologies, including the exquisitely chemosensitive germ cell tumors and primary central nervous system lymphomas, were intentionally omitted from this discussion because they do not represent the common challenges faced by chemotherapy in the treatment of brain metastases, as discussed in this chapter.

### Small Cell Lung Cancer

The incidence of developing symptomatic brain metastases is estimated to be ~50 percent, with approximately 10 percent of brain metastases identified at diagnosis and 40 percent identified later in the disease course. SCLC is typically very chemosensitive early in the disease course, regardless of the burden of initial disease (43). Although reported response rates vary widely, patients who have received little to no prior treatment appear to have brain metastases that are generally just as chemosensitive as the systemic disease. In contrast, patients who have received multiple prior treatments appear to have less chemosensitive brain metastases (44–46). Unfortunately, regardless of a patient's initial response to chemotherapy, the incidence of relapse, both systemically and in the brain, is high. Traditional chemotherapy agents include cisplatin, carboplatin, etoposide, irinotecan, topotecan, and others. The prevailing standard of care is a combination of platinum and etoposide. Newer chemotherapy agents and combinations have failed to provide superior results over this regimen, including in the prevention and/or control of brain metastases (47). Topotecan, recently FDA approved for the treatment of relapsed SCLC, is currently being evaluated for its use in the prevention and control of brain metastases. (The role of PCI in SCLC was discussed earlier in this chapter, in the section on micro-metastases.)

## Non-Small Cell Lung Cancer

It is estimated that ~20 percent of patients with non-small cell lung cancer (NSCLC) will develop brain symptomatic metastases within their lifetime (1). Brain metastases in NSCLC patients (as compared to brain metastases in SCLC) tend to occur later in the disease and with more than one lesion. NSCLC is also less chemosensitive than SCLC, even in patients who are naïve to radiation and chemotherapy. As in other histologies, response rates for chemotherapy are better early in the disease course, in the treatment naïve, and in the use of chemotherapies known to be chemosensitive in systemic NSCLC. Historically, clinical trials of chemotherapy for NSCLC brain metastases have not shown a significant improvement in outcomes over the use of radiation alone. Collectively, response rates for single and double chemotherapy agents range between 10 and 40 percent. Platinum-containing regimens and newer agents have the highest efficacy. In prospective trial of 43 treatment-naïve patients with NSCLC, the objective response rate to the combination of cisplatin and etoposide was 30 percent, and the median survival was 32 weeks (48). In other trials with treatment-naïve patients, platinums combined with paclitaxel, irinotecan, ifosfamide, vinorelbine, gemcitabine, and others have shown similar modest efficacy, with responses between 28 and 45 percent (48–51). When used singly, newer agents (such as topotecan) have unfortunately also only shown similar efficacy (52). When used in combination, newer agents (such as gemcitabine with irinotecan) have shown no improvement. In addition, these combinations have often shown increased toxicity. This was illustrated by the SWOG 0119 phase II trial performed in NSCLC patients with extensive disease and controlled brain metastases. Some received radiation to their systemic disease but none received chemotherapy. In this trial, 84 patients were treated with gemcitabine 1000 mg/m$^2$ and irinotecan 100 mg/m$^2$ on days 1 and 8 of a 21-day cycle, for a maximum of six cycles. The response rate of 32 percent was disappointing. The regimen was not well tolerated, with diarrhea occurring in 57 percent (grade 3/4, 18 percent) and other grade 3/4 toxicities occurring frequently: neutropenia (26 percent), anemia (10 percent), thrombocytopenia (8 percent), febrile neutropenia (5 percent), fatigue (11 percent), nausea (10 percent), and vomiting (8 percent) (53). Since the above clinical trial results were reported, translational research advancements and novel agents have provided new opportunities for use of chemotherapy in the multimodality care of brain metastases.

The modest efficacy of agents chosen for their chemosensitivity to systemic NSCLC has led researchers to evaluate agents by other criteria, such as CNS penetration. Given its excellent CNS penetration and promising efficacy in primary brain tumors, temozolomide has been evaluated in a variety of brain metastasis histologies, including NSCLC. In patients who developed metastases after previous WBRT, temozolomide has been relatively disappointing with responses ranging less than or equal to 20 percent (54–56). Furthermore, temozolomide has also been disappointing in patients who have not already had previous WBRT. This is exemplified by a phase II trial of NSCLC patient with multiple metastases who had not been previously treated with WBRT and who were randomized to either WBRT (30 Gy in 10 fractions) or temozolomide (200 mg/m$^2$ days 1 to 5 every four weeks). WBRT seemed to have a greater efficacy in controlling brain metastases recurrence at eight weeks than temozolomide alone (57).

However, the relatively disappointing results of temozolomide alone, whether before or after patients have received WBRT, stands in contrast to the improved radiographic responses seen when temozolomide and WBRT are concurrently administered to newly diagnosed NSCLC brain metastases patients. This was illustrated by a phase II study in which 52 patients were randomly assigned to WBRT either alone or with temozolomide. The overall response rate was significantly higher with the concurrent approach, 96 percent versus 67 percent (p =.017). Also of importance, fewer patients required corticosteroids two months after therapy, 67 percent versus 91 percent (18). Further investigations are ongoing.

Given that chemotherapy has not yet demonstrated significant treatment advances over surgery and radiation, alternative systemic agents continue to be evaluated. The identification of small molecule inhibitor agents as effective agents in lung cancer represents one of those strategies. Small molecule inhibitors, including the epidermal growth factor receptor (EGFR) inhibitors, are attractive for many reasons, including their frequent oral route of administration and absence of traditional toxicities, such as myelosuppression. Toxicities to the epidermal structures, including the skin, hair, nails and mucosa appears to be predominant, but are relatively manageable (58). Epidermal growth factor receptor inhibitors, including gefitinib and erlotinib, may have at least modest efficacy in NSCLC brain metastases. This was illustrated by a nonrandomized prospective phase II trial of 41 patients with newly diagnosed brain metastases treated with gefitinib. Twenty-seven percent experienced control of their disease, 4 patients with a partial response and 7 with stable disease (59). There is also evidence to suggest that EGFR inhibitor agents may demonstrate responses in recurrent NSCLC brain metastases (60). Although the role of EGFR inhibitors in NSCLC brain metastases is still evolving, review of the EGFR inhibitor literature that addresses both systemic disease and brain metastases reveals three apparently consistent themes. First, responses seem to be correlated to the presence of EGFR mutations, albeit they appear to be distinct mutations in different patient populations and disease types (61). Second, responses seem to be correlated to patients of Asian descent and patients who have never smoked (62). Third, responses seem to be correlated to the development of skin rash toxicity (63). These early suggestions of improved response and tolerability have prompted further evaluation, both with radiation or without, as well as with other chemotherapies or without. Similarly, further evaluations of EGFR inhibitors in the use of systemic NSCLC will require scrutiny to determine whether the brain is a sanctuary site, thus contributing to failure in the brain. This was at least suggested in a trial of 139 patients who experienced higher than average subsequent leptomeningeal metastases after receiving gefitinib (64). It will also be important to further explore whether certain histologies respond to EGFR inhibitors differently, something already seen in one large representative phase II trial of NSCLC, which suggested improved response of the histologic subtype of adenocarcinoma to gefitinib (65). Another small molecule inhibitor, a monoclonal antibody to the vascular endothelial growth factor receptor (VEGFR), bevacizumab, has been recently approved by the FDA for the treatment of advanced nonsquamous NSCLC. Anti-angiogenic agents, including bevacizumab, have demonstrated positive responses in primary brain tumors and peritumoral edema but have, unfortunately, demonstrated risks of intracranial hemorrhage and other deleterious vascular complications. Thus, clinicians are proceeding carefully with investigations of small molecule inhibitors in brain metastases.

Chemotherapy agents and small molecule inhibitors, with demonstrated chemo-sensitivity to systemic NSCLC, have been administered concurrently with radiation in an attempt to improve response. These agents include carboplatin, 5-fluorouracil, chloro-nitrosoureas, cisplatin, vinorelbine, teniposide, and others (21–23,66). Thus far, however, none of these systemically effective agents, when administered with concurrent radiation, have shown significant improvement outcomes over radiation alone.

## Breast Cancer

Breast cancer is the second most likely systemic malignancy to metastasize to the brain. Biologically, breast cancer has a high predilection for the brain, and is often the first site of relapse (67). This is at least partially secondary to the improved systemic control afforded by newer therapeutic combinations that results in patients living longer. This is also at least partially secondary to the reality that many systemic treatments currently used for breast cancer may not have significant CNS penetration. Both of these factors are well illustrated by the patients with HER-2 neu positive breast cancer who receive trastuzumab, a large antibody small molecule inhibitor of the Her-2 neu receptor, as part of a very efficacious multimodality regimen (68–70). Whether the documented increased incidence of breast cancer metastases in this population is reflective of longer survival afforded by this trastuzumab or, instead, trastuzumab's inability to penetrate the CNS, remains a controversial topic of investigation. Nonetheless, patients treated with this agent require adequate surveillance (71,72).

Breast cancer is one of the most chemosensitive solid malignancies. Chemotherapy agents proven efficacious to systemic breast cancer include taxanes, platinums, anthracyclines, antimetabolites, alkylating agents, vinorelbine and others. Although, these agents do not significantly penetrate the intact BBB, they have each demonstrated some degree of response in the setting of brain metastases. This suggests that the relative disruption of the BBB in the setting of brain metastases may allow a wider array of agents impact outcomes in the CNS. As with other histologies, responses to chemotherapy are better in those patients early in their disease course, in the treatment naïve, and in the use of agents known to be chemosensitive to systemic breast cancer. Numerous chemotherapy regimens have demonstrated objective responses, ~30 to 80 percent in the setting of newly diagnosed brain metastases, and in some cases leptomeningeal metastases. Common components of these regimens include cyclophosphamide, 5-flourouracil (5-FU), capecitabine (oral 5-FU pro-drug), methotrexate, vincristine, etoposide, cicplatin, carboplatin, topotecan, and others (25,48,73–79). When reviewed collectively, the responses are not superior to those when WBRT is utilized alone.

Moreover, in the setting of recurrent brain metastases, the responses of chemotherapies known to have efficacy in systemic breast cancer are even less impressive. Therefore, just as with other histologies, clinicians have turned toward agents known for their excellent CNS penetration. Temozolomide has been evaluated in recurrent breast cancer brain metastases. Unfortunately, responses to date have been disappointing, ranging from 0 to ~20 percent (55,80). Despite this early trial experience, temozolomide, given its ability to palliate the symptoms of brain metastases and its relative tolerance by older patients, may still have a role in treating this patient population (81–83). It addition, the role of temozolomide may also increase if its concurrent administration with other chemotherapy agents improves responses and/or palliation. The latter is suggested in a small phase I trial, where concurrent temozolomide and capecitabine were administered to breast cancer brain metastases patients until progression. Fourteen of the 24 were newly diagnosed, and 10 were recurrent and had received up to 3 prior chemotherapy regimens. Results included 18 percent objective response rate, 12 week median time to progression, and stable to improved neurocognitive function in those patients with stable disease or response (84).

Over the past decade, small molecule inhibitors have revolutionized the treatment of patients with breast cancer. Three of the most important small molecule inhibitors include trastuzumab, an IV humanized monoclonal antibody against the HER-2 receptor; bevacizumab, an IV monoclonal antibody against the vascular endothelial growth factor receptor (VEGFR); and lapatnib, an oral "dual-active" ERB-1 and HER-2 (ERB-2) tyrosine kinase inhibitor. Trastuzumab does not significantly penetrate the BBB, whereas both bevacizumab and lapatinib do. Although the complex causative factors are still being elucidated, the widely experienced phenomenon of increased brain metastases in patients given trastuzumab, has resulted in the increased use of lapatinib (70,85). Also effective in systemic HER-2 neu positive breast cancer, lapatinib appears both to penetrate the BBB and to have early promise in this patient population. In a phase II trial, 39 patients who developed brain metastases while on trastuzumab were administered lapatinib (750 mg twice daily), with 2 patients with a partial response, 1 with a minor response, and 5 with stable disease for several months (86). Lapatinib is currently FDA approved in combination with capecitabine in HER-2 positive breast cancer patients who require treatment and who have previously received taxane, trastuzumab, or anthracycline. Interestingly, in this sentinel study, fewer patients in the lapatinib group developed brain metastases as the first site of progression (11 versus 4) (87). Interest in lapatinib increased after this study was published and, currently, numerous trials are ongoing with lapatinib, alone in combination with other chemotherapies, in patients with HER-2 positive breast cancer brain metastases. The agent is also currently being evaluated with other small molecule inhibitors, including bevacizumab (88). Lapatinib promises to be an important tool in the treatment of HER-2 positive breast cancer metastases.

It is worth mentioning that brain metastases may also respond to endocrine therapy. Tamoxifen has been shown to achieve significant concentrations in brain metastases and several cases of response have been reported (89,90). Letrozole, an aromatase inhibitor, may have a similar effect (91).

## Melanoma

The incidence of melanoma is increasing at a rate greater than any other human cancer. Patients with melanoma have the 3rd highest predilection for the development of symptomatic brain metastases within their lifetime. Regardless of the location or burden of disease, melanoma is considered both relatively radioresistant as well as chemoresistant and is, therefore, very difficult to treat. Despite this, systemic agents are still used in the high-risk adjuvant, recurrent, or metastatic settings, either alone or in combination. These include interferon-alfa (INF-a), high-dose interleukin 2 (IL-2), dacarbazine (DTIC), platinums, and investigational agents, such as small molecule inhibitors (92). As with other histologies, response rates are highest for agents known to be chemosensitive in systemic melanoma and in the treatment naïve (48). Temozolomide was identified as a potential agent for melanoma brain metastases when clinical trials of its use in systemic melanoma reported less frequent failures in the brain (93). Dedicated trials followed. To date, temozolomide shows one of the most consistent responses as a single agent against melanoma brain metastases. As in this phase II study, sadly, overall objective response rate are only ~10 percent (94). The combination of temozolomide and thalidomide did not show any better response but did show increased toxicity, predominantly thromboembolic events and fatigue (95,96). A phase II observational trial of 62 previously untreated advanced melanoma patients, 8 of whom had brain metastases, the combination of docetaxel and temozolomide resulted in 3 of the 8 brain metastases partially responding (97). Other combinations, such as lomustine and temozolomide, both well known for their BBB penetration, have shown no activity in a similar patient population (98). Other chemotherapies have been evaluated in combination with biologic systemic agents. IL-2 and interferon-alfa are two biologic agents which have produced partial responses in systemic metastatic melanoma, including those with preexisting brain metastases. Their addition to cisplatin did not improve response in 14 such patients (99,100). Chemotherapy dose intensification has also proved an unsuccessful strategy to date. This is illustrated by a prospective, multicenter, open-label phase II trial of dose-intensified temozolomide. 45 asymptomatic patients with documented brain metastases (21 chemotherapy naïve and 24 with previous chemotherapy) were administered either temozolomide at 150 mg/m$^2$/day or at 125 mg/m$^2$/day during days 1 through 7 and 15 through 21 of a 28 day cycle. This biweekly schedule was fairly well-tolerated but showed ≤5 percent objective response rate in both the brain and systemic metastases (101). Current strategies being evaluated with temozolomide in melanoma brain metastases include the preselection of patients expected to have an increased response to temozolomide, such as those with a methylated-MGMT DNA repair enzyme, or the preselection of dosing schedules expected to prevent chemoresistance via MGMT-dependent mechanisms. Current strategies also include the concurrent administration of temozolomide and radiation expected to selectively circumvent DNA repair in metastatic cells. Despite the relatively disappointing results of early studies, clinical trials with temozolomide are still warranted in melanoma brain metastases, especially given that the alternative of radiation must be avoided in some patients and given that numerous temozolomide-based regimens have not yet been evaluated (102).

As with other histologies, attempts to improve the response rate led to the evaluation of temozolomide administered concurrently with WBRT. This is illustrated by one phase II trial of 35 unresectable melanoma brain metastases patients who had received 0 to 1 prior chemotherapies. 200 mg/m$^2$ of temozolomide was administered on days 1 to 5 every 28 days in all patients and was concurrently administered with some form of radiation (WBRT or SRS) in 22 of 35. In 34 evaluable responses, 1 was complete, 2 were partial, and 9 were stable disease. The median time to progression was 5 months, the median survival 8 months, and toxicities were similar to those seen when either was used alone (103). Other agents, selected for their excellent BBB penetration, such as nitrosureas (carmustine (BCNU), lomustine (CCNU), and fotemustine), have failed to provide response rates greater than ~15 better (104–106). This is illustrated by a phase III trial of patients with melanoma brain metastases, where fotemustine was administered concurrently with WBRT. This combination failed to improve the response rate or overall survival over WBRT alone, however, it did increase the median time to progression of subsequent brain metastases significantly (107). The alternative strategy of combining SRS ($\pm$ WBRT) with chemotherapy, such as temozolomide, for melanoma brain metastasis patients is being evaluated (108). In summary, the almost-epidemic increase in melanoma incidence worldwide, combined with its relative radioresistance and chemoresistance, underscore the pressing need for both innovative clinical trial design and participation. It is likely that chemotherapy will play an increasing role in the future multimodality treatments in melanoma brain metastases.

## Other Histologies

A few concepts regarding other histologies in brain metastases are worth mentioning. The consistent improvements in both local and systemic treatments in other systemic malignancies have directly resulted in an increased incidence of brain metastases in patients, as well. A few notable examples include colorectal, ovarian, prostate, and liquid malignancies (109–111). For the brain metastases occurring in these other histologies, there is less evidence regarding efficacious therapies, often only small case series or anecdotal experience. As with brain metastases in lung, breast and melanoma, the brain metastases in these other histologies typically have the best responses to chemotherapy early in the disease course, in the treatment naïve, and in the use of chemotherapies known to be chemosensitive in the systemic disease. The emergence of clinical trials dedicated to evaluating the efficacy of chemotherapy both in brain metastases and in specific histologies will hopefully yield effective evidence-based treatments in the near future.

## Future Directions

Brain metastases represent a tremendous burden on human society, whether measured by the devastation to an individual patient's quality of life or by the costs associated with a worldwide healthcare crisis. The past few decades been marked by the development of some of the tools necessary to relieve this burden with numerous new classes of systemic agents to test in brain metastases, as well as with the evolution of better preclinical models of representative challenges in brain metastases treatment in which to test them. Historically, the role of chemotherapy has been largely limited to use after local therapies have failed and has been limited to palliation instead of disease control. However, more recently, the role of chemotherapy is increasing in parallel with the advancements achieved with multimodality approaches.

The results of numerous multiinstitutional randomized trials will become available soon and will further define the role of various systemic chemotherapies used concurrently or sequentially with SRS, WBRT, and radiosensitizing agents. However, this chapter's review of chemotherapy in the care of brain metastases has highlighted areas where research achievements must occur if brain metastases are ever to become less burdensome in the future. A few examples of suggested research agendas follow:

- Research is needed for the prevention of cancer and the prevention of recurrence, including strategies with functional imaging (FDG-PET, MR-spect, tractography, etc.), biomarkers, PCI, systemic treatment for high-risk patients in the adjuvant setting, and defining optimal screening for occult disease.
- Research is needed for the improvement of delivery into the CNS of systemic agents, including strategies with anti-angiogenic agents, nanotechnology, BBB disruption via radiation, ultrasound, antibodies, or other systemic agents, or local delivery of agents via polymers, catheters or gels.
- Research is needed for the development of new systemic agents, including strategies with newer ways to circumvent the BBB via nanoparticles or osmotic agents, with agents designed to target chemotherapy-resistance pathways via gene mutations, efflux pumps or other mechanisms, and with novel discoveries via industry or translational researchers.
- Research is needed for the improvement of multimodality therapy, including strategies with chemotherapy combinations with other systemic agents and forms of radiation.

- Research is needed for the improvement of supportive care, including strategies with technologies to limit the area or severity of toxicity, with medicines to improve tolerance, and with rehabilitation approaches to maintain function.

- Research is needed for the improvement both of preclinical (translational) and clinical trial design, with strategies to separate new versus recurrent brain metastases, with mechanism-based and histology-specific analyses, and with the dedication to collect and analyze serial tissue specimens.

- Finally, research is needed for the improvement clinical trial endpoints that are meaningful both to patient and researcher, including strategies to better understand the true impact of brain met recurrence versus toxicities of therapies, with incorporation and validation of the following endpoints: neurocognitive function, neurologic function, quality of life, brain control, neurologic causes of death, and disability. When these areas of future research are reviewed collectively, it is quite apparent that the role of chemotherapy in the care of brain metastases will continue to strengthen and expand.

# References

1. Barnholtz-Sloan J, Sloan A, Avis F, et al. Incidence proportions of brain metastases in patients diagnosed (1973-2001) in the Metropolitan Detroit Cancer Surveillance System. *J Clin Oncol* 2004; 22: 2865–2872.
2. Schouten IJ, Rutten J, Huveneers HA, et al. Incidence of brain metastases in cohort of patents with carcinoma of the breast, colon, kidney, lung and melanoma. *Cancer* 2002;94:2698–2705.
3. Loeffler J, Barker F, Chapman P. Role of radiosurgery in the management of central nervous system metastases. *Cancer Chemother Pharmaco* 1999; 43: S11–S4.
4. Gavrilovic IT, Posner JB. Brain metastases: epidemiology and pathology, *J Neurooncol* 2005; 75:5–14.
5. Patchell RA. The management of brain metastases. *Cancer Treat Rev* 2003;29:533–540.
6. U.S. Census Bureau. http://www.census.gov. Revised: November 05, 2007.
7. Long DM. Capillary ultrastructure in human metastatic brain tumors. *J Neurosurg* 1979;51:53–58.
8. Zhang RD, Price JE, Fujimaki T, et al. Differential permeability of the blood-brain barrier in experimental brain metastases produced by human neoplasms implanted into nude mice. *Am J Pathol* 1992 Nov;141(5):1115–1124.
9. Gerstner ER, Fine RL. Increased permeability of the blood-brain barrier to chemotherapy in metastatic brain tumors: establishing a treatment paradigm *J Clin Oncol* 2007;25(6): 2306–2312.
10. Donelli MG, Zucchetti M, D'Incalci M. Do anticancer agents reach the tumor target in the human brain? *Cancer Chemother Pharmacol* 1992;30(4):251–260.
11. Lassman AB, DeAngelis LM. Brain metastases. *Neurol Clin* 2003; 21(1):1–23 vii.
12. Moscetti L, Nelli F, Felici A, et al. Up-front chemotherapy and radiation treatment in newly diagnosed non-small cell lung cancer with brain metastases: Survey by Outcome

Research Network for Evaluation of Treatment Results in Oncology. *Cancer* 2007;109(2):274–281.

13. DiStefano A, Yong Yap Y, Hortobagyi GN, et al. The natural history of breast cancer patients with brain metastases. *Cancer* 1979;44(5):1913–1918.

14. Agboola O, Benoit B, Cross P, et al. Prognostic factors derived from recursive partitioning analysis (RPA) of Radiation Therapy Oncology Group (RTOG) brain metastases trials applied to surgically resected and irradiated brain metastatic cases. *Int J Radiat Oncol Biol Phys* 1998;42:155–159.

15. Gaspar LE, Scott C, Rotman M, et al. Recursive partitioning analysis (RPA) of prognostic factors in three Radiation Therapy Oncology Group (RTOG) brain metastases trials. *Int J Radiat Oncol Biol Phys* 1997;37:745–751.

16. Gaspar LE, Scott C, Murray K, et al. Validation of the RTOG recursive partitioning analysis (RPA) classification for brain metastases. *Int J Radiat Oncol Biol Phys* 2000;47: 1001–1006.

17. Chang EL, Wefel JS, Maor MH, et al. A Pilot Study of neurocognitive function in patients with one to three new brain metastases initially treated with stereotactic radiosurgery alone. *Neurosurgery* 2007;60:277–283.

18. Antonadou D, Paraskeavaidis M, Sarris G, et al. Phase II randomized trial of temozolomide and concurrent radiotherapy in patients with brain metastases. *J Clin Oncol* 2002; 20:3644–3650.

19. Verger E, Gil M, Yaya R, et al. Temozolomide and concomitant whole brain radiotherapy in patients with brain metastases: A phase II randomized trial. *Int J Radiat Oncol Biol Phys* 2005;61(1):185–191.

20. Addeo R, Caraglia M, Faiola V, et al. Concomitant treatment of brain metastasis with whole brain radiotherapy [WBRT] and temozolomide [TMZ] is active and improves quality of life. *BMC Cancer* 2007;7:18.

21. Guerrieri M, Wong K, Ryan G, et al. A randomised phase III study of palliative radiation with concomitant carboplatin for brain metastases from non-small cell carcinoma of the lung. *Lung Cancer* 2004;46:107–111.

22. Ushio Y, Arita N, Hayakawa T, et al. Chemotherapy of brain metastases from lung carcinoma: A controlled randomized study. *Neurosurgery* 1991;28(2):201–205.

23. Robinet G, Thomas P, Breton JL, et al. Results of a phase III study of early versus delayed whole brain radiotherapy with concurrent cisplatin and vinorelbine combination in inoperable brain metastasis of non-small-cell lung cancer: Groupe Francais de Pneumo-Cancerologie (GFPC) Protocol 95-1. *Ann Oncol* 2001;12:59–67.

24. Stevens MF, Hickman JA, Langdon SP, et al. Antitumor activity and pharmacokinetics in mice of 8-carbamoyl-3-methyl- imidazo[5,1-d]-1,2,3,5-tetrazin-4(3H)-one (CCRG 81045; M & B 39831), a novel drug with potential as an alternative to dacarbazine. *Cancer Res* 1987;47:5846–5852.

25. Lassman AB, Abrey L E, Shah GD, et al. Systemic high-dose intravenous methotrexate for central nervous system metastases. *J Neurooncol* 2006;78(3):255–260.

26. Su YB, Sohn S, Krown SE, et al. Selective CD4+ lymphopenia in melanoma patients treated with temozolomide: A toxicity with therapeutic implications. *J Clin Oncol* 2004;22: 610–616.

27. Suh J, Stea B, Nabid A, et al. Standard whole brain radiation therapy (WBRT) with supplemental oxygen (O2), with or without RSR13 (efaproxiral) in patients with brain metastases: Results of the randomized REACH (RT-009) study. *Proc Am Soc Clin Oncol* 2004; 22:115S.

28. Komarnicky LT, Phillips TL, Martz K, et al. A randomized phase III protocol for the evaluation of misonidazole combined with radiation in the treatment of patients with brain metastases (RTOG-7916). *Int J Radiat Oncol Biol Phys* 1991;20:53–58.

29. haw E, Scott C, Suh J, et al. RSR13 plus cranial radiation therapy in patients with brain metastases: Comparison with the Radiation Therapy Oncology Group Recursive Partitioning Analysis Brain Metastases Database. *J Clin Oncol* 2003;21(12):2364–2371.

30. Phillips TL, Scott CB, Leibel SA, et al. Results of a randomized comparison of radiotherapy and bromodeoxyuridine with radiotherapy alone for brain metastases: Report of RTOG trial 89-05. *Int J Radiat Oncol Biol Phys* 1995;33:339–3348.

31. Patel R, Mehta M. Targeted Therapy for Brain Metastases: Improving the Therapeutic Ratio. *Clin Ca Res* 2007;13(6):1675–-1683.

32. Richards G, Khuntia D, Mehta M. Therapeutic management of metastatic brain tumors. *Critical Reviews in Oncology/Hematology* 2007;6:70–78.

33. Khuntia F, Mehta M. MG: A clinical review of a novel radio-enhancer for brain tumors. *Expert Rev Anticancer Ther* 2004;4:981–989.

34. Mehta MP, Rodrigus P, Terhaard CH, et al. Survival and neurologic outcomes in a randomized trial of motexafin gadolinium and whole-brain radiation therapy in brain metastases. *J Clin Oncol* 2003;21:2529-2536.

35. Meyers CA, Smith JA, Bezjak A, et al. Neurocognitive function and progression in patients with brain metastases treated with whole-brain radiation and motexafin gadolinium: Results of a randomized phase III trial. *J Clin Oncol* 2004;22:157–165.

36. Mehta MP, Gervais R, Chabot P, et al. Motexafin gadolinium (MGd) combined with prompt whole brain radiation therapy prolongs time to neurologic progression in non-small cell lung cancer (NSCLC) patients with brain metastases: Results of a phase III trial (abstract). *J Clin Oncol* 2006 ASCO Annual Meeting Proceedings Part I. 24;18S (June 20 Supplement).

37. Forouzannia A, Richards G M, Khuntia D, et al. Motexafin gadolinium: A novel radiosensitizer for brain tumors. *Expert Rev Anticancer Ther* 2007;7(6):785–794.

38. Fortin D, Gendron C, Boudrias M, et al. Enhanced chemotherapy delivery by intraarterial infusion and blood-brain barrier disruption in the treatment of cerebral metastasis. *Cancer* 2007;109(4):751–760.

39. Fortin D, Desjardins A, Benko A, et al. Enhanced chemotherapy delivery by intraarterial infusion and blood-brain barrier disruption in malignant brain tumors: The Sherbrooke experience. *Cancer* 2005;103(12):2606-2615.

40. Doolittle ND, Peereboom DM, Christoforidis GA, et al. Delivery of chemotherapy and antibodies across the blood-brain barrier and the role of chemoprotection, in primary and metastatic brain tumors: report of the Eleventh Annual Blood-Brain Barrier Consortium meeting. *J Neurooncol* 2007;81(1):81–91.

41. Slotman B, Faivre-Finn C, Kramer G, et al. EORTC Radiation Oncology Group and Lung Cancer Group Prophylactic Cranial Irradiation in Extensive Small-Cell Lung Cancer. *N Engl J Med* 2007;357(7):664–672.

42. Pugh TJ, Gaspar LE. Prophylactic cranial irradiation for patients with lung cancer. *Clin Lung Cancer* 2007;8(6):365–368.

43. Grossi F, Scolaro T, Tixi L, et al. The role of systemic chemotherapy in the treatment of brain metastases from small-cell lung cancer. *Crit Rev Oncol Hematol* 2001;37(1):61-67.

44. Postmus PE, Smit EF, Haaxma-Reiche H, et al. Teniposide for brain metastases of small-cell lung cancer: a phase II study. European Organization for Research and Treatment of Cancer Lung Cancer Cooperative Group. *J Clin Oncol* 1995;13:660–665.

45. Seute T, Leffers P, Wilmink JT, et al. Response of asymptomatic brain metastases from small-cell lung cancer to systemic first-line chemotherapy. *J Clin Oncol* 2006;24(13): 2079–2083.

46. Groen HJ, Smit EF, Haaxma-Reiche H, et al. Carboplatin as second line treatment for recurrent or progressive brain metastases from small cell lung cancer. *Eur J Cancer* 1993; 29A(12):1696–1699.

47. Lorusso V, Galetta D, Giotta F, et al. Topotecan in the treatment of brain metastases. A phase II study of GOIM (Gruppo Oncologico dell'Italia Meridionale). *Anticancer Res* 2006;26(3B):2259–2263.

48. Franciosi V, Cocconi G, Michiara M, et al. Front-line chemotherapy with cisplatin and etoposide for patients with brain metastases from breast carcinoma, nonsmall cell lung carcinoma, or malignant melanoma: a prospective study. *Cancer* 1999;85(7):1599–1605.

49. Fujita A, Fukuoka S, Takabatake H, et al. Combination chemotherapy of cisplatin, ifosfamide, and irinotecan with rhG-CSF support in patients with brain metastases from non-small cell lung cancer. *Oncology* 2000;59(4):291–295.

50. Cortes J, Rodriguez J, Aramendia JM, et al. Front-line paclitaxel/cisplatin-based chemotherapy in brain metastases from non-small-cell lung cancer. *Oncology* 2003;64(1):28–35.

51. Bernando G, Cuzzoni Q, Strada MR, et al. First-line chemotherapy with vinorelbine, gemcitabine, and carboplatin in the treatment from non-small cell lung cancer: A phase II study. *Cancer Invest* 2002;20:293–302.

52. Wong ET, Berkenblit A. The role of topotecan in the treatment of brain metastases. *Oncologist* 2004;9(1):68–79.

53. Akerley W, McCoy J, Hesketh PJ, et al. Gemcitabine and irinotecan for patients with untreated extensive stage small cell lung cancer: SWOG 0119. *J Thorac Oncol* 2007;2(6):526–530.

54. Dziadziuszko R, Ardizzoni A, Postmus PE, et al. Temozolomide in patients with advanced non-small cell lung cancer with and without brain metastases. A phase II study of the EORTC Lung Cancer Group (08965). *Eur J Cancer* 2003;39:1271–1276.

55. Abrey LE, Olson JD, Raizer JJ, et al. A phase II trial of temozolomide for patients with recurrent or progressive brain metastases. *J Neurooncol* 2001;53:259–265.

56. Giorgio CG, Giuffrida D, Pappalardo A, et al. Oral temozolomide in heavily pre-treated brain metastases from non-small cell lung cancer: phase II study. *Lung Cancer* 2005;50(2): 247–254.

57. Wagenius G, Brodin O, Nyman J, et al. Radiotherapy vs. temozolomide in the treatment of patients with lung cancer and brain metastases: A randomized phase II study (abstract). *J Clin Oncol* 2006 ASCO Annual Meeting Proceedings Part I. 24:18S (June 20 Supplement).

58. Galimont-Collen AF, Vos LE, Lavrijsen AP, et al. Classification and management of skin, hair, nail and mucosal side-effects of epidermal growth factor receptor (EGFR) inhibitors. *Eur J Cancer* 2007;43(5):845–851.

59. Ceresoli1 GL, Cappuzzo F, Gregorc V, et al. Gefitinib in patients with brain metastases from non-small-cell lung cancer: A prospective trial. *Ann Oncol* 2004;15:1042–1047.

60. Popat S, Hughes S, Papadopoulos P, et al. Recurrent responses to non-small cell lung cancer brain metastases with erlotinib. *Lung Cancer* 2006;56(1):135–137.

61. Shimato S, Mitsudomi T, Kosaka T, et al. EGFR mutations in patients with brain metastases from lung cancer: Association with the efficacy of gefitinib. *J Neurooncol* 2006;8: 137–144.

62. Hann CL, Brahmer JR. Who should receive epidermal growth factor receptor inhibitors for non-small cell lung cancer and when? *Curr Treat Options Oncol* 2007;8(1):28–37.

63. Chiu CH, Tsai CM, Chen YM, et al. Gefitinib is active in patients with brain metastases from non-small cell lung cancer and response is related to skin toxicity. *Lung Cancer* 2005;47(1):129–138.

64. Omuro AM, Kris MG, Miller VA, et al. High incidence of disease recurrence in the brain and leptomeninges in patients with non-small cell lung carcinoma after response to gefitinib. *Cancer* 2005;103:2344–2348.

65. Wu C, Li Y, Wang Z, et al. Gefitinib as palliative therapy for lung adenocarcinoma metastatic to the brain. *Lung Cancer* 2007;57(3):359–364.

66. Postmus PE, Haaxma-Reiche H, Smit EF, et al. Treatment of brain metastases of small-cell lung cancer: Comparing teniposide and teniposide with whole-brain radiotherapy-a phase III study of the European Organization for the Research and Treatment of Cancer Lung Cancer Cooperative Group. *J Clin Oncol* 2000;18:3400–3408.

67. van den Bent MJ. The role of chemotherapy in brain metastases. *Eur J Cancer* 2003 Oct;39(15):2114–2120.

68. Bendell JC, Domchek SM, Burstein HJ, et al. Central nervous system metastases in women who receive trastuzumab-based therapy for metastatic breast carcinoma. *Cancer* 2003; 97(12):2972–2977.

69. Tham YL, Sexton K, Kramer R, et al. Primary breast cancer phenotypes associated with propensity for central nervous system metastases. *Cancer* 2006;107(4):696–704.

70. Pestalozzi BC, Zahrieh D, Price KN, et al. Identifying breast cancer patients at risk for Central Nervous System (CNS) metastases in trials of the International Breast Cancer Study Group (IBCSG). *Ann Oncol* 2006;17(6):935–944.

71. Kirsch DG, Ledezma CJ, Mathews CS, et al. Survival after brain metastases from breast cancer in the trastuzumab era. *J Clin Oncol* 2005;23:2114–2116.

72. Duchnowska R, Szczylik C. Central nervous system metastases in breast cancer patients administered trastuzumab. *Cancer Treat Rev* 2005;31:312–318.

73. Boogerd W, Dalesio O, Bais EM, et al. Response of Brain Metastases from breast cancer to systemic chemotherapy. *Cancer* 1992;69:972–980.

74. Rosner D, Nemoto T, Lane WW. Chemotherapy induces regression of brain metastases in breast carcinoma. *Cancer* 1986;58:832–839.

75. Oberhoff C, Kieback DG, Wurstlein R, et al. Topotecan chemotherapy in patients with breast cancer and brain metastases: Results of a pilot study. *Onkologie* 2001;24:256–260.

76. Wang ML, Yung WK, Royce ME, et al. Theriault RL Capecitabine for 5-fluorouracil-resistant brain metastases from breast cancer. *Am J Clin Oncol* 2001;24(4):421–424.

77. Rogers LR, Remer SE, Tejwani S. Durable response of breast cancer leptomeningeal metastasis to capecitabine monotherapy. *J Neurooncol* 2004;6(1):63–64.

78. Siegelmann-Danieli N, Stein M, Bar-Ziv J. Complete response of brain metastases originating in breast cancer to capecitabine therapy. *Isr Med Assoc J* 2003 Nov;5(11):833–834.

79. Ekenel M, Hormigo AM, Peak S, et al. Capecitabine therapy of central nervous system metastases from breast cancer *J Neurooncol* 2007;85(2):223–227.

80. Trudeau ME, Crump M, Charpentier D, et al. Temozolomide in metastatic breast cancer (MBC): A phase II trial of the National Cancer Institute of Canada–Clinical Trials Group (NCIC-CTG). *Ann Oncol* 2006;17(6):952–956.

81. Christodoulou C; Bafaloukos D; Kosmidis P, et al. Phase II study of temozolomide in heavily pretreated cancer patients with brain metastases. *Ann Oncol* 2001;12(2):249–254.

82. Siena S, Landonio G, Baietta E, et al. Multicenter phase II study of temozolomide therapy for brain metastasis in patients with malignant melanoma, breast cancer and non-small cell lung cancer. American Society of Clinical Oncology 39th Annual Meeting, Chicago, Illinois, May 31–June 3, 2003. Abstract #407. *Proc Am Soc Clin Oncol* 2003;22:102.

83. Friedman HS, Evans B, Reardon D, et al. Phase II trial of temozolomide for patients with progressive brain metastases. American Society of Clinical Oncology 39th Annual Meeting, Chicago, Illinois, May 31–June 3, 2003. *Proc Am Soc Clin Oncol* 2003;22:102.

84. Rivera E, Meyers C, Groves M, et al. Phase I study of capecitabine in combination with temozolomide in the treatment of patients with recurrent brain metastases from breast carcinoma. *Cancer* 2007;107(6):1348–1354.

85. Errante D, Bernardi D, Bianco A, et al. Brain metastases in patients receiving trastuzumab for breast cancer. *Neurol Sci* 2007;28:52–53.

86. Lin NU, Carey LA, Liu MC, et al. Phase II trial of lapatinib for brain metastases in patients with HER2+ breast cancer (abstract). *J Clin Oncol* 2006;24:3S.

87. Geyer CE, Forster J, Lindquist D, et al. Lapatinib plus capecitabine for HER2-positive advanced breast cancer. *N Engl J Med* 2006;355(26):2733–2743.

88. Mayer EL, Lin NU, Burstein HJ. Novel approaches to advanced breast cancer: bevacizumab and lapatinib. *J Natl Compr Canc Netw* 2007;5(3):314–323.

89. Nicdcr, Salvati M, Cervoni L, et al. Prolonged stabilization of multiple and single brain metastases from breast cancer with tamoxifen: Report of three cases. *Tumori* 1993;79(5):359–362.

90. Lien EA, Wester K, Lonning PE, et al. Distribution of tamoxifen and metabolites into brain tissue and brain metastases in breast cancer patients. *Br J Cancer* 1991;63(4):641–645.

91. Madhup R, Kirti S, Bhatt ML, et al. Letrozole for brain and scalp metastases from breast cancer: A case report. *Breast* 2006;15(3):440–442.

92. Kirkwood JM, Strawderman MH, Ernstoff MS, et al. Interferon alfa-2b adjuvant therapy of high-risk resected cutaneous melanoma: The Eastern Cooperative Oncology Group trial EST 1684. *J Clin Oncol* 1996;14:7–17.

93. Sommers Y, Middleton M, Calvert H, et al. Effect of temozolomide (TMZ) on central nervous system relapse in patients with advanced melanoma (abstract). *Proc Am Soc Clin Oncol* 1999;18:531a.

94. Agarwala SS, Kirkwood JM, Gore M, et al. Temozolomide for the treatment of brain metastases associated with metastatic melanoma: a phase II study. *J Clin Oncol* 2004; 22(11):2101–2107.

95. Hwu WJ, Lis E, Menell JH, et al. Temozolomide plus thalidomide in patients with brain metastases from melanoma. *Cancer* 2005;103(12):2590–2597.

96. Krown SE, Niedzwiecki D, Hwu WJ, et al. Phase II study of temozolomide and thalido-mide in patients with metastatic melanoma in the brain: high rate of thromboembolic events (CALGB 500102). *Cancer* 2006;108(8):1883–1890.

97. Bafaloukos D, Gogas H, Georgoulias V, et al. Temozolomide in Combination With Docetaxel in Patients With Advanced Melanoma: A Phase II Study of the Hellenic Cooperative Oncology Group. *J Clin Oncol* 2002;20:420.

98. Larkin JM, Hughes SA, Beirne DA, et al. A phase I/II study of lomustine and temozolo-mide in patients with cerebral metastases from malignant melanoma. *Br J Cancer* 2007; 96(1):44–48.

99. Richards JM, Gale D, Mehta N, et al. Combination of chemotherapy with interleukin-2 and interferon-alfa for the treatment of metastatic melanoma. *J Clin Oncol* 1999;17:651.

100. Mousseau M, Khayat D, Benhammouda A, et al. Feasibility study of chemo-immunotherapy (Ch-IM) with cisplatin (CDDP) interleukin-2 (IL-2) and interferon alpha 2a (IFNa) on 14 melanoma brain metastases patients (pts) (abstract). *Proc Am Soc Clin Oncol* 1997;16:1773a.

101. Schadendorf D, Hauschild A, Ugurel S, et al. Dose-intensified bi-weekly temozolomide in patients with asymptomatic brain metastases from malignant melanoma: A phase II DeCOG/ADO study. *Ann Oncol* 2006;17(10):1592–1597.

102. Boogerd W, de Gast GC, Dalesio O. Temozolomide in advanced malignant melanoma with small brain metastases: Can we withhold Cranial Irradiation? *Cancer* 2007;109: 306–312.

103. Hofmann M, Kiecker F, Wurm R, et al. Temozolomide with or without radiotherapy in melanoma with unresectable brain metastases. *J Neurooncol* 2006;76(1):59–64.

104. Atkins, MB. The role of cytotoxic chemotherapeutic agents either alone or in combination with biological response modifiers. In: Molecular Diagnosis, Prevention and Therapy of Melanoma. Kirkwood, JK (Ed.). New York: Marcel Dekker, 1997. p.219.

105. Houghton AN, Legha S, Bajorin DF. Chemotherapy for metastatic melanoma. In: Cutaneous Melanoma, 2nd ed. Balch CM, Houghton AN, Milton GW, et al (Eds). Philadelphia: JB Lippincott. 1992, p.498.

106. Jacquillat C, Khayat D, Banzet P, et al. Final report of the French multicenter phase II study of the nitrosourea fotemustine in 153 evaluable patients with disseminated malig-nant melanoma including patients with cerebral metastases. *Cancer* 1990;66:1873.

107. Mornex F, Thomas L, Mohr P, et al. A prospective randomized multicentre phase III trial of fotemustine plus whole brain irradiation versus fotemustine alone in cerebral metas-tases of malignant melanoma. *Melanoma Res* 2003;13(1):97–103.

108. Samlowski WE, Watson GA, Wang M, et al. Multimodality treatment of melanoma brain metastases incorporating stereotactic radiosurgery (SRS). *Cancer* 2007;109(9):1855–1862.

109. Sundermeyer ML, Meropol NJ, Rogatko A, et al. Changing patterns of bone and brain metastases in patients with colorectal cancer. *Clin Colorectal Cancer* 2005;5:108–113.

110. Pectasides D, Pectasides M, Economopoulos T. Brain metastases from epithelial ovarian cancer: a review of the literature. *Oncologist* 2006;11:252–260.

111. Tay SK, Rajesh H. Brain metastases from epithelial ovarian cancer. *Int J Gynecol Cancer* 2005;15(5):824–829.

# 8

# Supportive Care
## Controlling Symptoms of Brain Metastasis and Diminishing the Toxicities of Treatment

Stephanie E. Weiss

The clinical management of patients who have metastatic brain disease is currently undergoing a major reevaluation. Previously thought of as an imminently terminal event, metastatic brain disease, due to major improvements in therapy in recent years, can now often be viewed as a chronic condition. This change of view and the resulting change in approach has been driven not only by the improved therapies for brain metastasis described elsewhere in this book, but also by better therapies for systemic metastasis that are resulting in improved survival in general.

Increasing survival among patients with metastatic brain disease has, in turn, altered how we interact with patients and prescribe therapy because greater consideration needs to be given to quality of life issues. As a result, the treatment of patients with metastatic disease, including those who have brain metastases, has become increasing complex. While we may hope to cure in a small percentage of patients, our hope for many is simply to prolong life. However, we should try to ensure that all patients remain symptom free and in good health. We have many treatment modalities to help us in this task, but, as is so often the case in medicine, beneficial effects are often achieved at the risk of inducing unwanted side effects.

This chapter will review important aspects of supportive care for patients with brain metastasis. The use of steroid therapy for cerebral edema and symptoms of mass effect is necessary for many patients, although careful management is required as these steroids themselves have toxicities that may have devastating effects on quality of life and health. Other topics include acute side effects and long-term risks of radiotherapy, fatigue, seizure prophylaxis, radionecrosis, thrombotic events, and cognitive effects of therapy.

# Dexamethasone for Mass Effect and Neurologic Symptoms

If there are no symptoms to indicate the presence of cerebral edema, dexamethasone therapy is not routinely indicated. This often applies to patients who are incidentally diagnosed with brain metastases during a screening magnetic resonance imaging (MRI).

Neither is treatment inevitably indicated in asymptomatic patients who are about to undergo a course of radiation therapy to the brain. This situation requires careful clinical assessment, given the range of possible complications that are associated with steroid therapy. The radiation oncologist has a significant role in deciding whether steroids should be given to asymptomatic patients in advance of treatment.

## Complications of Steroid Therapy

*Gastrointestinal upset* We routinely place all patients taking steroids on gastrointestinal (GI) prophylaxis with an H2 blocker or proton-pump inhibitor. Though there is a paucity of data supporting their routine use in the prevention of GI bleeds in outpatients, the risk of the medication is generally sufficiently low. Thus, unless expressly contraindicated, we feel their use is worthwhile, given the devastating effects of a bleed. They also minimize gastrointestinal upset and symptoms of heartburn associated with steroids.

*Sleep disturbance* This is one of the most common, immediate, and troublesome side effects of steroid therapy. Typically, patients complain that they are unable to sleep through the night or that they awaken several times during the night. The consequence of such disturbance in sleep pattern, daytime fatigue, can be difficult to distinguish from cancer or treatment related fatigue. Daytime naps are frequently resorted to but rarely compensate for lost nighttime sleep.

In the short term, a drug in the sedative-hypnotic class (such as zolpidem) may help such patients considerably. Although anxiolytics such as lorazapam can have sedating effects, they less frequently provide restorative sleep. The choice of drug is determined by patient response. If a patient is already on one or more sedating drugs, it is often effective and safer to merely adjust dosage of one of these drugs to achieve the desired result.

In the intermediate term, a potentially effective strategy is to favor reduction of the evening doses of steroid during the "taper." Steroid need may be lowest during periods of rest, and a somewhat asymmetric tapering favoring the evening doses may help restore a normal sleep cycle. As always, tapering should be undertaken in such a way as to keep the patient symptom free. If symptoms reappear, they will typically do so within 48–72 hours. Patients should be alerted that symptoms occurring days after a reduction in steroid dose may, in fact, be a result of the taper.

Fortunately dexamethasone is somewhat flexible with respect to dosage scheduling. Doses can be scheduled to avoid having to awaken the patient from sleep. Thus the patient may receive medication early morning, midday, evening, and finally, prior to sleep even though this regime is not strictly evenly divided over the 24-hour period. Indeed, if the patient requirements can accommodate it, consider scheduling the last dose of the day a few hours earlier than bedtime as this may contribute to better rest at night. As usual, steroids should be taken with food to prevent gastrointestinal upset. The patient should also receive an H2-blocker, proton pump inhibitor, or other prophylaxis against possible GI inflammation.

*Increased appetite* Steroid-induced overeating is a normal feature of treatment that will disappear when the drug is tapered off. This is one side effect that can even be considered to be beneficial in this group of patients who are often anorexic or cachectic secondary to the disease or to therapy. Despite the apparent benefit, steroids should not be used as an appetite stimulant and should only be prescribed if there is an indicated need, i.e., to control side effects of edema. The other effects of long-term dexamethasone therapy, including immunosuppression and significant proximal myopathy, can reduce quality of life and can be life threatening. Cancer-related anorexia and fatigue should be treated by agents other than dexamethasone (this issue will be addressed later). Patients should also be reassured that the dexamethasone-induced increased appetite will return to normal when therapy is ended.

*Personality changes* One of the more disturbing effects of steroid both for patients and their families is the possibility that steroids might result in personality changes. Such a change may manifest itself as an increase in energy or even euphoria. Some patients may even resist discontinuation of medication because of the loss of their new-found well being. More usually however, the sorts of symptoms that are associated with steroid treatment are not desired either by patient or family and include agitation and anxiety. Fortunately, these symptoms are typically mild to moderate and are easily managed conservatively, simple patient education often being sufficient to enable a patient to understand what is happening and to cope with it. Where necessary a low dose of an anxiolytic such as Lorazapam may help and can be tapered in parallel with the steroid taper. Caution is always necessary when prescribing this drug with other similarly acting drugs or with drugs that can cause respiratory depression.

In rare cases, personality changes can be severe. Patients may develop manic behavior, psychosis, and even suicidal or homicidal tendencies. These problems can occur even in patients who have no previous history of psychiatric disorder. While infrequently seen, when such symptoms develop in patients receiving dexamethasone, they should be treated as emergencies requiring urgent psychiatric consultation, possible antipsychotic medication, and taper of dexamethasone as tolerated.

On the other hand, despite their ability to cause such psychiatric symptoms, steroids are not necessarily contraindicated in patients who have a prior history of psychiatric disorders. The treating clinician should exercise increased vigilance in such patients, closely monitoring behavior; even invoking the assistance of a psychiatrist to ensure that onset of such symptoms is detected early.

What alternative treatment can be given to such patients if they have to stop dexamethasone therapy? We have found that if for any reason patients cannot tolerate dexamethasone, a COX-2 inhibitor may be substituted with some chance of success (1,2). COX-2 inhibitors block prostaglandin synthesis and control the side effects associated with edema, often with surprising effectiveness. However the efficacy of these agents has not been rigorously studied and documented. Moreover, these agents have been associated with cardiovascular complications in recent studies, something that needs to be factored into any decision to use them.

*Steroid induced diabetes mellitus* Steroids are diabetogenic. Blood glucose levels should be monitored once treatment is commenced. Patients should be educated about the symptoms associated with hyperglycemia, frequent urination, polydipsea, polyphagia and, in the longer term, visual changes. If it is expected that steroids will be administered over a long period of time, antiglycemic agents may be indicated. In the short term, such agents are usually not necessary unless the blood sugar level exceeds 250 mg/dl.

*Steroids and infection: increased steroid demand* The immunosuppressive and anti-inflammatory effects of steroids increase susceptibility to infection, which in turn increases a patient's steroid demand. The clinician should have a high index of suspicion of infection should a patient complain of symptoms referable particularly to the urinary or respiratory tract.

Infection may lead indirectly to worsening of the neurological symptoms that prompted the initial diagnosis of brain metastasis. Alternatively symptoms of elevated intracranial pressure may develop and progress. Under either of these circumstances, the possible role of intercurrent infection should be considered in the differential and should be included in the work-up along with other suspicious causes. In addition to appropriate antibiotic therapy for the infection, the patient will also require a temporary increase in steroid dose to compensate for increased demand associated with the stress of the infection.

*Steroids and infection: polymorphonuclear cell (PMN) demargination* Dexamethasone treatment is commonly associated with an elevation in the peripheral white blood cell count due to the fact that it down-regulates cell membrane-associated adhesion molecules and prevents polymorphonuclear cells from leaving the circulation. This phenomenon may be confused with infection induced neutrophilia. On the other hand, it is possible that a patient who has increased PMN count due to steroid intake may also have an infection. In short, the PMN count is not as reliable an indicator of infection in patients who are receiving steroids and should not be relied on excessively. The presence of a PMN increase in the CBC with a shift to the left (i.e. *bandemia*) however, should alert the physician to the likelihood of infection. In general, low threshold of suspicion for infection needs to be maintained in the setting of patients on steroids and physicians should routinely question patients to elicit early warning signs. If infection is suspected it should be aggressively investigated. Chest X-ray, urinalysis with culture and sensitivity, and blood cultures are all indicated.

If a craniotomy has been performed, possible operative site infection should be excluded. The risk of wound infection or even meningitis persists for weeks postoperatively. A computed tomography (CT) or MRI may be helpful in making the diagnosis. If infectious (or carcinomatosis) meningitis is suspected, this will require, in addition to scans, a lumber puncture, which should be performed with extreme caution to avoid the possibility of herniation.

*Steroids and infection: Fever* Fever in a patient who is receiving dexamethasone should *always* raise a red flag. Ordinarily steroids antagonize the development of fever as part of their anti-inflammatory effect so the absence of a fever does not rule out the possibility of serious infection in a patient. Therefore the presence of even a minor elevation of a patient's baseline temperature should prompt immediate aggressive workup to determine the cause. Especially important are urinary tract infections, respiratory tract infection, pneumonia (including pneumocystis carinii pneumonia or PCP), extensive or systemic candidiasis or, in the postcraniotomy setting, brain abscess, meningitis, or wound infection at the operative site, which as noted earlier, may occur even many weeks after surgery.

One other thing to be aware of is that the interpretation of a chest X-ray may be compromised in patients receiving steroids because their anti-inflammatory actions may reduce the expected fluid exudation into the alveolar spaces. Repeat imaging might be necessary to monitor such patients.

*Pneumocystis carinii pneumonia* Pneumocystis carinii pneumonia (PCP) is relatively common in immunosuppressed individuals and can be difficult to recognize. Patients on dexamethasone for a few weeks may develop PCP, especially (though not exclusively) if they are also elderly. As well as facilitating infection, steroids also impair the body's defenses against the causative agent. The anti-inflammatory effect of steroids is used therapeutically to offset symptoms associated with alveolar edema and improve respiration in patients with PCP.

Thus, dexamethasone use over the intermediate term both renders the patient susceptible to, and masks the symptoms of, life-threatening PCP. Chest-X-ray may be deceptively benign in appearance and should be repeated in the setting of any unexplained fever in a patient on dexamethasone.

The suspicion for PCP should be heightened in the classic scenario of worsening fever or the development of respiratory symptoms in a patient whose dexamethasone dosage is being actively tapered, typically after a period of use of more than 3 weeks. Fever may be an early warning sign in this setting as respiratory symptoms may not appear until later because the anti-inflammatory action of the steroids may still be intact. Possible respiratory tract infection in this setting should be treated as an emergency, and a negative chest X-ray should be always be viewed with some skepticism. Empiric treatment may be warranted.

It is generally a good idea to consider PCP prophylaxis in all patients who are on steroids for more than a month, especially for those over the age of 60.

Alternately, patients on steroids for over 1 month may be routinely screened for their CD4+ count and prophylaxis started if the number falls below 200 cells/µL. Trimethoprim-sulfamethoxazole (TMP-SMX) double strength, three times per weeks is a very good standard regimen. If a patient does not tolerate sulfa drugs or has any contraindication to bactrim, then Dapsone, Atovaquone or monthly Pentamadine treatments can be considered.

*Steroids and thrush* Patients receiving whole-brain radiation and patients on steroids are both at risk for oral candidiasis (thrush). Such patients typically complain of taste changes and/or a sore throat. Thrush can typically be managed with fluconazole tablets, or an oral nystatin rinse. Clotrimazole troches are also useful. If left untreated, a patient's well-being may be compromised. Oral intake of nutrition and fluids is typically decreased, which can lead to profound decompensation. In severe cases, the infection can become extensive or systemic. Its typically a manageable complication and patients on steroids and receiving whole-brain radiation should be routinely screened for candidiasis.

*Drug allergies: Mask and flare* One should always consider the possibility that the development of pyrexia in a patient who is receiving Dexamethasone may be caused by a drug allergy. This is especially important in patients who have newly established metastatic disease to the brain as these are frequently placed on several new agents that may induce such a reaction.

In the early stages of treatment, an allergic response to one or other of these new medications may be masked if there is concomitant treatment with steroids. It is during the steroid taper phase that such an allergic response may become evident for the first time as the body regains its ability to mount an inflammatory response. Initial symptoms usually include a uticaria or maculopapullar rash on the extremities, chest, and trunk. The lesions may become confluent. Swelling, dyspnea, or fever may also occur. It is important to recognize these symptoms for what they are as they may worsen and even become life threatening if administration of the offending agent is not stopped.

While many drugs can induce an allergic response, two in particular are prone to do so in patients who are being treated for metastatic brain disease. These are trimethoprim-sulfamethoxazole (TMP-SMX) and phenytoin (Dilantin.) It is estimated that up to 25 percent of patients with brain tumors develop an immunologic reaction to Dilantin. Despite this, it is still the favored drug when there has been a seizure, and it is also favored by neurosurgeons as prophylaxis in the postoperative setting due to the ease with which blood levels can be measured to ensure maintenance of therapeutic levels during the acute period.

Failure to recognize and treat drug allergies may lead to serious morbidity and mortality, including Stevens-Johnson syndrome. If allergy is suspected, the likely offending agents should be removed immediately and substituted with alternative drugs (such as Keppra for treatment of seizures and Dapsone instead of Bactrim). Antihistamines may be administered or steroid dosage may be temporarily increased if indicated for moderately severe symptomatic reactions. Emergency care and hospital admission may be necessary for those who develop severe reactions.

*Steroid related swelling and deep venous thrombosis (DVT)* Retention of water and swelling of the extremities is not an uncommon side effect of longer-term steroid treatment. It is obviously important to differentiate between such swelling and that which may be associated with deep venous thrombosis. Classically DVT causes unilateral lower extremity swelling while steroid edema is typically bilateral. Despite this rule of thumb, we know that cancer patients in general and patients with brain tumor or those who are postoperative in particular have a very high risk for DVT. The clinician should therefore have a very high index of suspicion when dealing with any lower limb swelling, and lower extremity Doppler ultrasound should be performed to exclude DVT. Bilateral DVT is certainly not uncommon and can even occur in a patient who already has steroid-related lower extremity edema.

Treatment will involve anticoagulation, if not contraindicated by any other feature of the patient's condition—including the brain metastases themselves. Input by oncologists is valuable in the evaluation of the role of anticoagulants in this setting. If anticoagulant therapy is contraindicated, then a Greenfield filter may be an alternative. In our experience, inferior vena cava filters in this clinical circumstances are associated with a significant incidence of thrombosis (due to the malignancy related hypercoaguable state) and consequent need for anticoagulation anyway. For this reason, we favor anticoagulation in the absence of any special contraindications.

A diagnosis of DVT should always be followed by assessment of the patient to exclude pulmonary embolism. Any new or unexplained respiratory symptoms should certainly include pulmonary embolism in the differential diagnosis. A dry cough is often a subtle sign. Shortness of breath at rest or on moderate activity, pleuritic chest pain, or low oxygen saturation are all signs that should raise suspicion.

If DVT is ruled out as a cause, steroid-related lower extremity edema can typically be managed conservatively with TEDs stockings and elevation of the legs. If such conservative measures are not successful diuretics may be considered.

## Common Long-Term Effects of Dexamethasone

Despite their effectiveness in treating edema-related symptoms, steroid treatments should be tapered as soon possible. There are many long-term complications of dexamethasone treatment. Below we will consider some of the more serious.

*Proximal myopathy* Patients who receive steroid therapy over a period of several weeks to several months are at high risk for debilitating proximal myopathy. They may initially note onset of fatigue while climbing stairs or find that it is difficult to rise from the sitting position and that they must leverage themselves up by the armrests. These symptoms will get progressively worse with time if a steroid taper is not started, and they are not alleviated by the usual exercises designed to arrest muscular atrophy. Not only do these symptoms cause mental distress associated with recognition of deteriorating physical capacity, they also may lead to other serious side effects. A patient may eventually become wheelchair bound, and this increasing immobility increases risk of infection and DVT.

Steroid dosage should be tapered as aggressively as possible in these patients consistent with their clinical status. Supportive education should also be provided to patients. They should be encouraged to take regular exercise, a regime that also has the advantage of empowering patients with a sense of control over their own well-being. Patients who are in good physical condition often find that a stationary bicycle is a beneficial and safe means of exercise.

*Cushing's syndrome* With prolonged steroid use, patients will develop Cushing's syndrome with the classic "moon facies" and "buffalo hump." The severity and rate of development of this syndrome is dose dependent and varies from patient to patient.

Cancer patients often have to deal with issues regarding body image caused either by the disease itself or by treatment. Surgery, radiation, and chemotherapy can all affect physical appearance. Alopecia, a consequence of whole-brain radiation, is a very striking reminder to patients of their new dependent status, one that is immediately obvious to all. The cushingoid appearance that results from prolonged steroid therapy is similarly obvious but is a side effect that cannot be masked by a remedy as simple as a hair prosthesis. It is also a visual reminder that the other effects of steroid therapy already alluded to above (immunosuppression, anti-inflammatory effect, diabetogenic effect etc) are progressing unseen beneath the surface.

*Adrenal insufficiency* As steroid dosages are reduced to relatively low levels during taper, patients may complain of onset of severe fatigue and general malaise. These may be a consequence of steroid-induced adrenal insufficiency caused by feedback inhibition of adrenocorticotropic hormone (ACTH) production by the pituitary gland. The resulting atrophy of the adrenal cortex requires time to recover. The answer to this problem is to slow down the rate of taper as the daily dosage level approaches "replacement" level (approximately 1 mg po Dexamethasone bid). If problems persist, endocrinology consultation may be helpful.

*Other side effects*

Rarely, a fine tremor may develop in patients who receive dexamethasone. This fortunately reverses when the drug is discontinued. All that is required in this situation is to rule out more serious neurologic problems as a cause of the tremor.

Skin complications include delayed healing, thinning of skin due to the catabolic effects of steroids, and easy bruising. Patients may note an increase in facial hair and acne. Again, assurance that these conditions are likely to improve is usually all that is required.

Avascular necrosis of bone is a rare and serious complication. It is often heralded by the onset of join pain. Osteopenia, another consequence of the catabolic effects of steroids, is a more insidious bone problem.

In patients who cannot tolerate steroids or who have problems during the withdrawal phase, Celecoxib, a COX-2 inhibitor that inhibits prostaglandin synthesis, may be used to control side effects associated with cerebral edema. However Celecoxib and other cox-2 inhibitors may increase the risk of myocardial infarction and of cerebrovascular events. These side effects seem to be dose and duration dependent. The risk-benefit ratio needs to be considered. Patients with sulfa allergies should not take these agents.

## Short-Term Effects of Radiation Therapy for Brain Metastasis

*Fatigue* Radiation, and indeed even the presence of brain metastases them-selves, are both frequently associated with profound chronic fatigue. Classically, patients will find themselves becoming tired earlier in the day than usual, reviving well with restorative sleep. This problem generally becomes more noticeable once radiation therapy has begun, especially if whole-brain radiation is administered. Symptoms may even get progressively worse for a week or so after the course of treatment has ended. Symptoms are quite vari-able in severity, multifactorial in etiology, and unpredictable.

Patients should be warned in advance of treatment that this might occur and, if it does, the best treatment is symptomatic management, including scheduled naps and good general sleep hygiene. This, of course, can be con-founded by another side effect of the steroids noted earlier, their tendency to induce insomnia. Judicious use of sleep-hypnotic agents such as Zolpidem may help.

If refractory fatigue lasts for a long period after the course of therapy has ended, stimulants may be considered. We prefer modafinil (or Armodafinil), which seem to have minimal effect on the seizure threshold in patients with brain tumors (3). These drugs are typically well tolerated, agitation and headache being the main side effects. Other useful agents that can potentially help combat radiation-induced fatigue include Methylphenidate (Ritalin) (4,5) and Donepezil (Aricept) (6).

*Seizure* Patients should only be placed on anti-epileptic medication if they have had a seizure and prophylactic treatment upon diagnosis has not been proven to be helpful and exposes patients to risk of toxicity (7). Phenytoin (Dilantin) is the drug of first choice and has the very important advantage that blood levels can be monitored accurately. However, it is estimated that up to 25 percent of patients who have a brain tumor will develop a sensitivity or allergy to this drug. This may first become obvious as steroid therapy is being tapered as noted above. Stevens-Johnson syndrome, a rare but serious reaction, can also occur.

Many patients who are initially treated with these agents will therefore require an alternative. Levetiracetam (Keppra) is generally well tolerated and effective in seizure control. Unfortunately it is not possible to monitor blood levels so doses have to be titrated symptomatically. The most common side effects are fatigue and depression.

The input of a neurologist or neurosurgeon is desirable when initiating or changing anti-epileptic therapy.

If a patient has had a seizure, caused either by a brain lesion or subsequent to craniotomy, he or she may be especially prone to radiation-related "irritation" and should stay on prescribed antiseizure medications during and immediately after the course of radiation therapy. In patients who have not had a history of seizures, whole-brain radiation does not typically increase the risk of such an occurrence.

*Skin irritation*  Radiation treatment of brain metastases may induce mild to moderate skin erythema typically over the cranium and from the forehead down to the brow. The effect is especially obvious in very fair skinned persons of northern European extraction. Symptoms may be minimized by the simple expedient of instructing patients to avoid using harsh lotions or chemicals or alcohol containing products on their skin immediately before and after treatment.

Patients should be clearly instructed to make sure that their skin is clean, dry, and free from any topical products when they present for radiation therapy sessions. Even thin layers of lotions or creams can create a bolus effect wherein radiation dose is "pulled" toward the skin, exacerbating skin irritation.

In the expectation of skin irritation, and as a precautionary measure, we favor Biafine topical emulsion and recommend application even before symptoms manifest. Eucerin, an over-the-counter preparation, can also be helpful. The daily application of these products can be deferred until after treatment if this is scheduled for early in the day. If treatment is scheduled for later in the day these preparations may be applied early in the morning but should be completely removed prior to treatment and reapplied afterwards.

As might be expected, skin irritation is less pronounced in darker skinned persons but may still be quite significant, and pigmentation akin to tanning is more common. Nevertheless, even if irritation is not particularly prominent, Biafine can also help soothe dryness and peeling and promote healing of skin.

During the treatment period, other harsh chemicals should be avoided on the skin of the head. Hair dyes and straightening and other cosmetic hair agents should be avoided. Baby shampoo is recommended.

*Hair loss*  Alopecia is an integral part of whole-brain treatment. It usually becomes noticeable in the second week of treatment and onset may be sudden. Patients should be well prepared for this sometimes devastating side effect, which is a visible reminder of their status as cancer patients. Patients often comment that they are not only shocked at their appearance when they view themselves in the mirror but that the reaction of others to their plight can be equally disturbing. Judicious use of scarves, hats, or hair prostheses (which may be covered by health insurance) may be helpful.

Unfortunately, recovery of hair growth cannot be guaranteed in all patients; sometimes hair loss is permanent. Hair growth on the vertex is usually slowest, due to the physics of the beam arrangement. Prior chemotherapy can also adversely influence regrowth.

Even when everything is favorable, hair recovery after radiation therapy is a slow process, and it typically takes about 3 months before substantial regrowth begins. Topical agents such as minoxidil might help although there is a paucity of data supporting this.

New protocols with intensity modulated radiotherapy (IMRT) and tomotherapy are being investigated to see if dose to the hair follicles can be decreased so as to minimize alopecia without adversely effecting treatment of parenchymal disease. However these techniques are investigational only at this point. Older techniques such as a "scalp block" have generally been ineffective in achieving their objective while putting the patient to a risk of inadequate treatment.

*Ear symptoms* The skin of the ear, like irradiated skin elsewhere, is likely to become inflamed. Observations made earlier in respect to skin problems also apply here. Occasionally, patients will complain of ear "stuffiness" during treatment, a condition believed to be caused by mild radiation-induced inflammation. This will resolve in time, but an infectious etiology should be ruled out. Otic steroids may be tried, but we feel they are of minimal benefit.

## Neurological Symptoms Arising During Treatment

Deterioration of a neurologic deficit in patients undergoing radiation for brain metastasis is worrying but may be the result of radiation-induced edema rather than progression. Small exacerbations of presenting symptoms are usually due to edema associated with the radiation treatment or with tapering of steroid dosage (or both). Other possibilities should be considered if symptoms do not respond to an incremental increase in steroid dosage, if new neurological symptoms appear, if there are any symptoms that might indicate increased intracranial pressure, or if there is a sudden or severe decompensation. In all of the above circumstances, infection (systemic or local, not necessarily neurologic) should be excluded as already discussed.

Bleeding into an intracranial metastasis may be an emergency situation, and it can be diagnosed with a noncontrast enhanced CT scan. Melanoma, renal cell carcinoma, and thyroid cancer metastases are at particularly high risk of bleeding, however most cases are seen among lung and breast cancer patients because these are the most common intracranial metastases treated. Indeed, any metastatic lesion in the brain should be considered a bleeding risk.

Brain tumor patients who are on nonsteroidal anti-inflammatory drugs (NSAIDs) or anticoagulants are especially at risk. Many patients are on drugs such as Lovenox or Warfarin due to cancer related co-morbidities such as DVT or pulmonary embolus. The benefit of these drugs has to be weighed against the very real risk that they may cause intralesional bleeding in the brain metastases. Neurosurgery consultation can be very helpful in such situations.

New neurological manifestations caused by wound infection at a craniotomy site, intracranial abscess, or infectious meningitis can be excluded by careful examination of the craniotomy site and a head scan. A lumber puncture may be necessary. Leptomeningial carcinomatosis should also be considered as a possible cause of unexplained or refractory neurological symptoms.

## Concomitant Chemotherapy

The blood brain barrier limits exposure of the brain to chemotherapeutic substances so that most agents have a negligible therapeutic effect on brain metastases. Nevertheless, these agents should be administered with caution when radiotherapy is being administered to the brain as blood brain barrier penetration may be sufficient to cause toxic radiosensitization that can exacerbate both the acute and the long-term side effects of radiation. Accordingly, the use of concurrent chemotherapy with radiation should be restricted to protocol or experienced specialists.

## Long-Term Risk of Radiation Treatment of Brain Metastasis

### Cognitive effects of whole-brain radiation
Some confusion surrounds the subject of long-term cognitive effects of whole brain radiation therapy (WBRT). It is

well known that radiation to the brain in children, particularly in those younger than seven years of age, can result in the emergence of serious and measurable cognitive defects, an effect that seems to be both dose and volume dependent (8). The effect of radiation to adult brains on cognition, although generally agreed to be real and sometimes substantial, is less well documented. Management strategies have not been well tested (10).

The problem is further confused by an important study published in the late 1980s in which severe late cognitive deficits were found in patients treated with whole-brain radiation for metastasis (11). However, these patients were treated with dose fraction schemes that are now no longer used, and in fact, these schedules were abandoned in large measure because of this study. Indeed, the same study demonstrated low risk for severe long-term effects with the dose fractionation schemes used in the modern era. Subsequent studies have demonstrated that the risk of significant neurocognitive decline and dementia is modest but real (8,9).

Nevertheless there are real long-term neuro-cognitive effects to consider for some patients who receive whole-brain radiation. The incidence and extent of neurocognitive deficit in adults resulting from whole-brain radiation seems to be related, at least in part, to the underlying health of the brain microcirculation.

Patients who already suffer from microvascular disease (diabetic patients, hypertensive subjects, patients who have a history of stroke or cardiovascular disease, patients who have dyslipidemias, and even those who are merely elderly) appear to be at greater risk of more serious long-term cognitive effect from WBRT. For this reason, it is somewhat paradoxical that it is often the younger, healthier patients for whom we express concern over the long-term effective of whole-brain radiation.

Cognitive deficits may manifest themselves as short-term memory loss often described by patients as "senior moments," such as misplacing keys, forgetting on which level they parked their car at a garage, or a tendency to repeat a conversation. Such symptoms are readily managed by simple measures such as keeping "to-do" lists and other simple behavioral modifications. Very rarely do cognitive changes become significantly debilitating in the absence of progressive central nervous system (CNS) disease or more global deterioration.

For patients felt to be at risk for significant predisposing cerebral vascular disease, alternative modalities to WBRT may be considered. Focal radiotherapy or radiosurgery alone with deferment of whole-brain treatment may be reasonable. This decision must be made with an experienced radiation oncologist.

Long-term cognitive changes following WBRT are likely to be irreversible and, if severe, may not be amenable to the behavioral modification techniques mentioned above. If cerebrovascular health can be optimized with medical management in such patients (i.e., statins or blood pressure lowering drugs if appropriate), it may help mitigate cognitive decline.

*Normal pressure hydrocephalus* In the absence of any definitive data in the modern radiation era, we are of the opinion that radiation to the brain may increase the likelihood of developing normal pressure hydrocephalus (NPH), especially in patients who have impairment of their cerebral microcirculation. Apart from its association with radiation therapy, NPH is now recognized to be underdiagnosed in the general populace. The cause of isolated NPH is unknown but one theory suggests that it is related to impaired microvascular health. The classic triad of presenting symptoms are increasing cognitive impairment, "magnetic" or shuffling gait, and urinary incontinence. Symptoms such as these are frequently ignored in elderly patients, seen merely as components of the ageing process, or misdiagnosed as elements of Alzheimer's disease or simple dementia. Examination of sequential MRIs of the brain will often reveal a subtle increase in size of the ventricles in these patients.

It is important to diagnose NPH because in a significant percentage of patients this disorder may be reversible. Diagnosis involves a brief hospital stay and a therapeutic lumbar drain trial conducted by a physician experienced in this procedure. If symptoms temporarily improve, a diagnosis of NPH is made, and the physician may discuss the definitive placement of a therapeutic ventricular-peritoneal or lumbar-peritoneal shunt. The risks and benefits of shunting should be carefully considered before proceeding.

*Stroke* Patients who have received WBRT for brain metastases may be at increased risk for stroke. This is likely to be due to the changes of the microvasculature of the brain caused by the radiation. Treatment in these patients may be complicated by the fact that anticoagulation therapy may be contraindicated because of the risk of bleeding into residual metastasis.

*Imaging changes* Radiation induced leucoencephalopathy may be seen in patients who are monitored with serial MRI after whole brain radiation. Changes in the white matter of the brain are best appreciated on FLAIR weighted images and should be differentiated from lesion-related edema.

Such imaging changes in and of themselves do not require intervention unless asymptomatic.

Occasionally, following WBRT for metastatic brain disease, lesions may remain relatively stable in size and patients should be evaluated to determine if radiosurgery (which affords superior control of local disease) is appropriate. If lesions increase in size following WBRT (either due to increasing tumor mass or concomitant edema), the patient should be further investigated by the appropriate oncologist. Radiosurgery is a standard of care in the subpopulation of patients but also may be used palliatively in others.

Radionecrosis is not typical after WBRT in the absence of radiosurgery, but it should be considered as a differential diagnosis in patients whose lesions enlarge after treatment. Investigation may include functional imaging to help differentiate necrosis from progressive disease, but this is often not definitive. A low threshold of suspicion for progressive disease should be made in patients with enlarging lesions in the absence of radiosurgery as this radiation toxicity is uncommon with fractionated radiation. The development of new lesions should prompt referral back to the appropriate oncologist (radiation oncologist, neurosurgeon or medical oncologist).

*Rare side effects* Treatment side effects due to the effect of WBRT on normal brain structures can occur but are rare at currently accepted dosing levels. The dose tolerance of critical structures in the brain is an important consideration. Current dosing of whole-brain radiation is low enough to make visual problems, sensory or motor deficit, or brain stem dysfunction all exceedingly rare in this setting. Unless the patient has received radiosurgery or the dose of radiation that was administered deliberately exceeded the conventional dose, other causes should be sought for such symptoms if they arise.

Unless there has been a prior positive history, radiation rarely precipitates seizures. When they do occur they usually result from the treatment-induced irritation of the underlying lesion and are not usually attributable to the radiation per se.

Radiation-induced tumors are rare in any patient and especially in patients who receive treatment for brain metastases, given the latency of the effect. The most common radiation-induced tumor in this setting is a meningioma, typically an indolent tumor that requires treatment only if symptomatic. High-grade or malignant meningiomas may also arise as may other malignant tumors such as gliomas or sarcomas, but the possibility that such unfortunate outcomes might arise is greatly outweighed by the certainty of the outcome should brain metastases be left untreated.

# Patients Receiving Radiosurgery

In recent years, stereotactic radiosurgery (SRS) has emerged as a very useful technique in the treatment of some patients who have brain metastases. This is a noninvasive technique in which the patient receives a high dose of radiation targeted tightly to the lesion. The treatment is completed on a single day. Advantages include enhanced preservation of neurocognitive functions and prolonged survival in some patient populations.

Radiosurgery can be performed either as a stand-alone treatment or as an adjunct to WBRT. Many factors are taken into consideration in coming to a decision as to which modality to use, and these factors include the number of lesions to be treated, a patient's performance status, control of extracranial disease, and a patient's age. There are several different commercial brands of equipment and modes of delivery of SRS (gamma knife, CyberKnife, Novalis, linear-accelerator based). Some involve the temporary placement of a rigid frame on the patient to aid beam localization, others involve the implantation of targeting fiducials, or thermoplastic masks. In the vast majority of patients who have brain metastases, any of these technologies will be effective.

## *Acute Side Effects of SRS*

The incidence of significant side effects in patients who receive SRS is low. In preparation for the procedure, patients are routinely prescribed Dexamethasone and, if treatment is above the tentorium, anti-epileptic drugs. This prophylactic regime is comparable to, and modeled on, that used in patients who undergo invasive surgery and is practice based. This regime is not typically used in patients who receive WBRT. Steroids are tapered off as tolerated and anti-epileptic agents are typically tapered after two weeks if there is no history of seizure. Patients may experience the side effects associated with these drugs as previously discussed.

Transient nausea or headache related to the procedure is uncommon and minimized with the routine use of anti-emetics the day of treatment. Persistent or worsening headache, nausea, or vomiting or other symptoms that might indicate increasing intracranial pressure should receive prompt attention.

Alopecia and skin irritation are restricted to those areas where the beams converge and are usually minimal.

Treatment induced local edema may cause presenting symptoms to flare up in the days and weeks after treatment. If symptoms are mild and there is no indication that there might be infection, patients can be treated with a short course of dexamethasone therapy, which can usually be tapered over a period of around two weeks.

Persistent difficulty in withdrawing steroids or if symptoms get worse or if new symptoms appear, including systemic symptoms, should signal the possibility that other complications have arisen, such as intracranial bleeding, infection (local or systemic), severe edema, or even herniation. All of these should be ruled out. Ideally the treating physician, radiation oncologist, and neurosurgeon should all contribute to the management of such cases.

## Long-Term Effects of Radiosurgery: Radionecrosis

Radionecrosis is the most frequent complication of SRS in the months to years following treatment. Several factors are believed to contribute to this condition.

Tumor-cell death induces an inflammatory response with cytokine production, which may in turn induce an inflammatory response that can affect surrounding normal brain tissue. Secondly, although targeting of the radiation dose is highly focused, there is nevertheless some unavoidable exposure of surrounding normal tissue.

The dosimetry of radiosurgery is best understood as analogous to dropping a stone in a pond. The large "splash" at the point of impact of the stone when it hits the water represents the radiation dosage to the lesion, and the ripples that emanate from the epicenter correspond to radiation dose to normal tissues around the lesion. Just as the ripples become progressively weaker as they progress outwards, so also does the dosage of radiation that normal tissues receive in SRS. Even though the dose gradient outside of the lesion is steep (inversely related to the square of the distance), the dose to normal tissue is never zero and obviously this can contribute to normal tissue damage.

Radionecrosis is not often symptomatic. The main problem posed by this complication occurs during the posttreatment phase when the clinician seeks to determine if therapy has been successful on follow-up MRI. It can be difficult to distinguish between regions of radionecrosis and regions of tumor recurrence on MRI scans. Both may present as an increase in the size of the lesion, increased enhancement when gadolinium is administered, or worsening surrounding edema. A significant proportion of patients may have treatment related imaging changes. Bland imaging changes related to treatment may easily be confused with local tumor recurrence and therefore should be a realistic consideration for many patients with changes confined to the treated region and surroundings (12). Repeat MRI imaging can help, and further evaluation with modalities such as MRI spectroscopy, thallium scan, or a dedicated positron emission tomography (PET) scan of the brain may be useful. There is no consensus yet as to which of these modalities is superior to the others. The decision about which to use depends on the experience of the facility performing the investigation. In any event, a neuroradiologist who has been thoroughly briefed on the patient's clinical history should review the case.

It is critical to differentiate between necrosis and progressive disease. The latter may require intervention, including possible further radiation treatment, even if asymptomatic; the former may be monitored conservatively if asymptomatic or medically managed if symptomatic. The importance of arriving at the correct diagnosis is heightened by the fact that further radiation to a site of radionecrosis will inevitably aggravate the existing problem. If symptomatic, necrosis can be managed in the short and intermediate term with steroids which can treat the associated inflammation, usually the cause of symptoms. Patients who develop a combination of tumor progression *and* radionecrosis provide a difficult challenge in both the interpretation of the MRI imaging and in designing an appropriate treatment regime.

Other management options for patients who develop radionecrosis include surgical intervention. The use of hyperbaric oxygen treatments (13,14) is an unproved treatment that can be attempted in patients with unresectable tumors or those who are felt to be medically inoperable although there is not clear evidence of efficacy. Anticoagulant therapy has not been proven to be effective and may be risky in patients with brain metastasis. More recently, bevacizumab has been under investigation for this purpose (15).

To complicate matters, the symptoms that are associated with area of radionecrosis mimic those that are caused by a progressive lesion. The symptoms will vary depending on the region of the brain that is involved. Contralateral weakness may accompany a motor strip lesion, and difficulties with balance and gait characterize a cerebellar lesion. Seizures may accompany supratentorial lesions, however treatment with anti-epileptic agents is usually not required unless there has been a prior history of such attacks. As noted earlier these agents are used as prophylaxis at the time of the SRS procedure itself.

## Long-Term Risk of Radiosurgery: Possible Destruction of Vital Structures

High dose radiation therapy can damage the sensitive optic nerves, optic chiasm, or the brain stem if these structures are close to the targeted lesion. Damage by radionecrosis to these structures is best prevented by careful pre-treatment evaluation of the safety and appropriateness of the radiosurgery by an experienced team that includes a radiation oncologist and a neurosurgeon who specialize in radiosurgery.

If there is a concern about dose to these structures, fractionated stereotactic boosts can be delivered to protect normal tissue. Avastin (16,17), Pentoxiphyline, and vitamin E (17) have all been used to treat radiation-induced retinopathy and other side effects but their effectiveness is not clear.

## After Craniotomy

Surgical resection of a single brain metastasis has been shown to yield superior survival to radiotherapy. Surgery may also be beneficial for patients who have received radiation therapy if they have a large or symptomatic lesion and if symptoms do not respond to steroid therapy.

Postcraniotomy patients should be monitored carefully to detect side effects of common medications including anti-epileptics and steroids. They should also be monitored to detect early DVT or pulmonary embolism. Local or systemic infections can also be problematic in this group of patients, particularly if they are on steroids. Infection at the operation site or meningitis can manifest themselves deceptively late in the postoperative course and should be considered even after several weeks if suggestive signs or symptoms appear.

## Carcinomatosis

A word about leptomeningeal carcinomatosis merits inclusion in this discussion. Seeding of the leptomeninges is not uncommon and usually has a poor prognosis. However, several factors play into prognostication, including the histology of the primary tumor. Patients who have breast cancer metastases, for example, can have a relatively long survival with a good quality of life even within the setting of leptomeningeal disease.

The diagnosis of leptomeningeal carcinomatosis is often made when new neurologic symptoms arise or when discovered by imaging or by analysis of the cerebrospinal fluid. Cranial nerve deficits are particularly suggestive of carcinomatosis but are not pathognomonic for cerebrospinal fluid (CSF) spread. The patient may present with classical meningitis symptoms, nuchal rigidity, photophobia, headache, and nausea.

Where leptomeningeal carcinomatosis is suspected, an MRI evaluation is of value in making the diagnosis in about 50 percent of cases in the hands of a skilled neuroradiologist. Enhancement along the cranial nerves, a parenchymal pattern of disease around the sulci, or the presence of dural lesions are all suspicious features. Increased vascularity and "sugar coating" of the folia of the cerebellum are more definitive findings. CSF examination also is diagnostic in only about 50 percent of cases.

Radiation treatment for leptomeningeal disease is less successful than that used for discrete parenchymal mets. Whole-brain radiation can help symptomatically in about 50 percent of cases and may even retard progression. Chemotherapy either orally, IV or intrathecally (IT) is also disappointing in the treatment of the leptomeningeal spread of solid tumors. Caution should be taken if intrathecal therapy is considered as a high level of toxicity may occur if this is done in conjunction with brain radiation. This is particularly true with the use of IT-methotrexate.

Although leptomeningeal disease puts the whole cranial spinal axis at risk, craniospinal irradiation is rarely recommended. This treatment has a high morbidity and does not usually offer either durable control or palliation. Focal treatment to individual symptomatic or bulky lesions in the spine is reasonable and can be effective. Side effects of such treatments reflect the region treated (e.g., there may be GI upset if the lesion treated is at that level of the spinal cord).

## Summary

As with so many other cancer patient populations, the prognosis for patients who develop metastatic lesions in the brain can range from excellent to very poor. There are many treatment options, some more appropriate to certain situations than to others. The disease process and the treatments on offer are associated with symptoms and side effect that can almost always be managed to prolong life and well being. Physicians who deal with these patients should be aware of the common issues that face patients with metastatic brain disease and of the many therapeutic options that are available to help them.

# References

1. Khan RB, Krasin MJ, Kasow K, Leung W. Cyclooxygenase-2 inhibition to treat radiation-induced brain necrosis and edema. *J Pediatr Hematol Oncol* 2004; 26(4):253–255.

2. Portnow J, Suleman S, Grossman SA, Eller S, Carson K. A cyclooxygenase-2 (COX-2) inhibitor compared with dexamethasone in a survival study of rats with intracerebral 9L gliosarcomas. *Neuro Oncol* 2002;4(1):22–25.

3. Kaleita TA, Wellisch DK, Cloughesy TF, Ford JM, Freeman D, Belin TR, Goldman J. Prediction of neurocognitive outcome in adult brain tumor patients. *J Neurooncology* 2004;67(1-2):245–253.

4. Butler JM Jr., Case LD, Atkins J, Frizzell B, Sanders G, Griffen P, Lesser G, McMullen K, McQuellon R, Naughton M, Rapp S, Stieber V, Shaw EG. A phase III double blind, placebo-controlled prospective randomized clinical trial of d-threo-methylphenidate HCL in brain tumor patients receiving radiation therapy. *Int J Radiat Oncol Biol Phys* 2007;69(5): 1496–1501.

5. Weitzner MA, Meyers CA, Valentine AD. Methylphenidate in the treatment of neurobehavioral slowing associated with cancer and cancer treatment. *J Neuropsychiatry Clin Neurosci* 1995;7(3):347–350.

6. Shaw EG, Rosedhal R, D'Agostino RB Jr., Lovato J, Naughton MJ, Robbin NE, Rapp SR. Phase II study of donepazil in irradiation brain tumor patients: Effect on cognitive function, mood, and quality of life. *J Clin Oncol* 2006;24(9):1415–1420.

7. Glantz MJ, Cole BF, Forsyth PA, Recht LD, Wen PY, Chamberlain MC, Grossman SA, Cairncross JG. Practice parameter: anticonvulsant prophylaxis in patients with newly diagnosed brain tumors. Report of the Quality Standards Subcommittee of the American Academy of neurology. *Neurology* 2000;54(10):1886–1893.

8. Mulhern RK, Merchant TW, Gajjar A, Reddick WE, Kun LE. Late neurocognitive sequelae in survivors of brain tumours in childhood. *Lancet Oncol* 2004;5(7):399–408.

9. Meyers CA, Smith JH, Bezjak A, Mehta MP, Liebmann J, Illidge T, Kinkler I, Caudrelier JM, Eisenberg PD, Meerwaldt J, Siemers R, Carrie C, Gaspar LE, Curran W, Phan SC, Miller RA, Renschler MF. Neurocognitive function and progression in patients with brain metastases treated with whole-brain radiation and motexafin gadolinium: results of a radnomized phase III trial. *J Clin Oncol* 2004;22(1):157–165.

10. Butler JM, Rapp SR, Shaw EF. Managing the cognitive effects of brain tumor radiation therapy. *Curr Treat Options Oncol* 2006;7(6):517–523

11. DeAngelis LM, Delattre JY, Posner JB. Radiation-induced dementia in patients cured of brain metastasis. *Neurology* 1989;39(6):798–796.

12. Belohlavek O, Simonova G, Kantorova I, Novotny J, Liscak R. Brain metastases after stereotactic radiosurgery using the Leksell gamma knife: Can FDG PET help to differentiate radionecrosis from tumour progression? *Eur J Nucl Med Mol Imaging* 2003;30(1): 96–100.

13. Leber KA, Eder HG, Kovac H, Anegg U, Pendl G. Treatment of cerebral radionecrosis by hyperbaric oxygen therapy. *Stereotact Funct Neurosurg* 1998;70 Suppl 1:229–236.

14. Feldmeier JJ, Hampson NB. A systematic review of the literature reporting the application of hyperbaric oxygen prevention and treatment of delayed radiation injuries: An evidence-based approach. *Undersea Hyperb Med* 2002; 29(1):4–30.

15. Gonzalez J, Jumar AJ, Conrad CA, Levin VA. Effect of bevacizumab on radiation necrosis of the brain. *Int J Radiat Oncol Biol Phys* 2007;67(2):323–326.

16. Finger PT, Chin K. Anti-vascular endothelial growth factor bevacizumab (avastin) for radiation retinopathy. *Arch Opthalmol* 2007;125(6):751–756.

17. Delanian S, Lefaix JL. Current management for late normal tissue injury: Radiation-induced fibrosis and necrosis. *Semin Radiat Oncol* 2007;17(2):99–107.

# 9

# Radiosurgery for Spinal Tumors

Ori Shokek

Lawrence R. Kleinberg

The principals of radiosurgery are now being applied to spinal metastasis with the goal of further improving quality of life, protecting central nervous system function, and potentially increasing survival. Improving technology and increased understanding of the natural history of spinal metastasis are driving this line of investigation and may change disease management, just as occurred with brain metastasis management. A landmark trial, described below, has definitively demonstrated that aggressive local management substantially improves outcome. Compared with intracranial disease, where the skull may be simply immobilized and the brain tumor is fixed in relation to the skull, there were substantial challenges related to reproducibly positioning the patient, maintaining immobility, and aligning the treatment with respect to tumor, which may be abutting the spinal cord itself. Today, improved imaging, including improved magnetic resonance imaging (MRI) scanners and process MRI to computed tomography (CT) scan fusion (overlay), have allowed more accurate delineation of tumor, and more recently, technology has become available to precisely target spinal lesions with radiation.

## Historical Aspects of Radiotherapy for Spine Metastases

In operable patients with spinal metastases with spinal cord compression, decompressive surgery followed by external beam radiotherapy (EBRT) constitute optimal treatment for neurologic function. The well-publicized randomized trial reported in 2005 by Patchell et al. (1) assigned patients with spinal metastases causing spinal cord compression at a single area of the spinal cord to surgery followed by radiotherapy (at a dose schedule of 30 Gy in 10 fractions) versus radiotherapy alone (same dose schedule). An early stopping rule was met at an interim analysis, when it was observed that surgery plus radiotherapy was superior in terms of patient ability to walk after treatment (84 percent versus 57 percent) and also superior with respect to the length of time that patients retained the ability to walk (122 days versus 13 days). Thirty-two patients who entered the study unable to walk fared significantly better with surgery plus radiotherapy (RT) in terms of regaining the ability to walk (62 percent versus 19 percent). Other endpoints significantly favoring surgery in conjunction with RT included the reduced need for corticosteroids and opioid analgesics.

Although this trial demonstrates the utility of surgery in addition to RT for patients with spine metastases and spinal cord compression, patients with metastatic cancer who are operable represent a select subgroup. Invasive surgery is not feasible for many patients with a terminal metastatic cancer diagnosis; for them, RT alone is used. Furthermore, the benefit of surgery with RT over RT alone is established in the setting of spine metastases with spinal cord compression per se, whereas RT alone is standard for patients without spinal cord compression who require treatment for pain, cauda equina compression, or radicular symptoms.

A variety of RT dose schedules have been used to treat spinal metastases. Rades et al. (2) retrospectively reported on 1,304 patients irradiated between 1992 and 2003 with several established schedules: 8 Gy in one fraction, 20 Gy in five fractions, 30 Gy in ten fractions, 37.5 Gy in 15 fractions, and 40 Gy in 20 fractions. Motor function improved in 26 percent to 31 percent of patients, and posttreatment ambulatory rates were 63–74 percent in the different dose schedule groups, without significant differences among them. However, in-field recurrences were significantly more common after 8 Gy in one fraction and 20 Gy in five fractions than with the other dose schedules (the number of patients with in-field recurrence in each RT dose schedule group were 34/261, 33/279, 12/274, 10/233, and 12/257, respectively). Randomized trials of different radiotherapy schedules for painful osseous metastases (not necessarily of the spine) have similarly observed that 8 Gy in one fraction is initially equally efficacious to more protracted dose schedules whose total dose is higher but that the latter are more efficacious in terms of long-term control of pain or the need for re-irradiation (3–7).

The RT dose schedules used in the above retrospective and prospective studies reflect a conservative approach to the palliative treatment of metastatic cancer patients, where the need to avoid RT-associated morbidity is extremely important. Specifically, avoiding iatrogenic myelopathy is paramount, and indeed it is rarely or never observed with these established dose schedules (2). The tolerance of the spinal cord is well studied. The total doses resulting in 0.1 percent, 1 percent, and 50 percent myelopathy rates in primates were observed to be 52 Gy, 59 Gy, and 76 Gy, respectively, when given in daily fractions of 2.2 Gy each (8). A modest volume effect has been observed, with higher rates seen when longer segments of the spinal cord are irradiated using a given dose schedule (9).

Those RT dose schedules in which the total dose is given using fractions ranging between 1.5 and 3 Gy daily reflect "standard fractionation." "Alternative fractionation" refers to schedules that employ larger daily fractions ('hypofractionation'), and there is currently a growing body of literature regarding single-fraction treatment. Single-fraction animal irradiation data for spinal cord tolerance have demonstrated a 50 percent paresis dose of 21–22 Gy in rats, and there appears to be a steep dose-paresis relationship, with a paresis threshold dose of approximately 19.5–20 Gy and a 100 percent paresis dose of approximately 21.5–23 Gy (10), observed by multiple researchers (11).

## Motivation for the Development of Spine Radiosurgery

In conventional radiotherapeutic management of spinal metastases, dose is commonly delivered to the spinal target by means of a single custom-shaped beam directed posteroanteriorly or by a pair of oppositely directed beam (the first posteroanterior, the second anteroposterior), resulting in undesired irradiation of organs anterior to the spine, such as the heart, liver, esophagus, and bowel. Cardiac side effects typically take many months to years to manifest and are therefore uncommonly experienced by metastatic cancer patients whose life expectancy is limited. Hepatic toxicity is also not usually experienced, as the typical arrangement of beams spares sufficient hepatic volume. In contrast, esophageal and bowel mucositis are experienced acutely with RT, but the resultant odynophagia, nausea, vomiting, and loose stools are usually mild and transient in metastatic cancer patients undergoing palliative spinal RT. Motivation nevertheless remains to limit the side effects of therapy and optimize quality of life. Minimizing the number of treatment visits is also important in this regard.

These considerations provide the motivation for single-fraction or hypofractionated spine radiosurgery, in which the total dose of radiation is delivered in a single or a few daily high-dose fractions. This is achieved using multiple beams, directed from multiple angles, which conformally converge upon the spinal target and limit dose to surrounding organs. Recent advances in computerized treatment planning and in image-guided delivery has enabled the development of radiosurgical techniques. As dosimetric accuracy in planning and delivery has been refined, radiosurgery treatments can now preferentially give dose to the spinal tumor while sparing the spinal cord itself (12). This treatment modality thus has the potential for dose-escalation, leading to more effective treatment of spine metastases as well as re-irradiation of spinal metastases that have failed prior to conventional RT or primary irradiation of unresectable primary tumors of the bony spine, such as Ewing sarcoma and osteosarcoma, for which the high total RT doses required for long-term local control exceed the threshold for myelopathy when delivered with conventional RT techniques (13–15). There is also the opportunity for treatment of epidural or intramedullary spinal cord tumors (16).

## Contemporary Results with Radiosurgery

While conventional RT is still viewed as standard therapy and continues to be commonly administered, several institutions that have adopted radiosurgery have accumulated large numbers of patients and have reported their outcomes. Gerszten et al. reported the University of Pittsburgh's prospective experience with 500 lesions treated in 393 patients to a mean dose of 20 Gy (range, 12.5–25 Gy). Treatment was delivered using the CyberKnife device, a linear accelerator mounted on a robotic arm. Among the 500 lesions, 31 percent were irradiated for the first time, and 69 percent were treated with radiosurgery after failing prior conventional RT (with dose schedules ranging from 30 Gy in 10 fractions to 35 Gy in 14 fractions). With a median follow-up interval of 21 months, long-term pain improvement was observed in 86 percent of patients, and long-term tumor control was observed in 90 percent of lesions treated with radiosurgery as the primary modality and in 88 percent of lesions treated with radiosurgery following conventional RT failure. Among 32 cases with progressive neurologic deficits prior to treatment, 84 percent experienced clinical improvement (17). The same group published results in the subset of spinal metastases, specifically in patients with lung carcinomas, with the majority (80 of 87) treated after failing prior conventional RT (30 Gy in 10 fractions to 35 Gy in 14 fractions). Mean radiosurgery dose was 20 Gy (range, 15–25 Gy).

Eighty-nine percent showed long-term pain improvement, and long-term radiographic tumor control was observed in all patients. Follow-up was short (median 12 months, range 6–40 months), reflective of the lifespan of metastatic lung carcinoma patients (18). Jin et al. reported technical aspects of the Henry Ford Hospital's radiosurgery experience regarding 270 lesions (none previously irradiated) treated in 196 patients using a Novalis radiosurgery system with a traditional gantry-mounted linear accelerator. Treatment was given in a single fraction, with a median dose of 14.8 Gy (range, 10–18 Gy). Clinical follow-up data were available for 49 patients, among whom pain relief was observed in 85 percent (12).

Reports regarding fractionated dose schedules are less abundant, with smaller numbers of patients treated. Yamada et al. (19) reported a heterogenous experience with 35 patients treated at Memorial Sloan-Kettering Cancer Center, 21 for spinal metastases and 14 for primary spinal tumors. For those previously irradiated, the mean prior conventional RT dose was 30 Gy in 10 fractions, and the radiosurgery median dose was 20 Gy in 5 fractions (range 20–30 Gy). For those not previously irradiated, the median dose was 70 Gy (range 59.4–70 Gy). The authors observed palliation from pain, weakness, or paresthesias in more than 90 percent of the patients. Local control was 75 percent in previously irradiated patients and 81 percent in those not previously irradiated.

## Spinal Cord Dosimetry and Myelopathy

Myelopathy has been reported uncommonly, both in patients who have received radiosurgery as the first treatment and in those who received radiosurgery following failed conventional RT. In Gerszten et al.'s experience with lung carcinoma patients, none experienced myelopathy. Cervicothoracic lesions' mean and median cord doses were both 9 Gy (range 4–12 Gy), and the mean and median cord volumes exceeding 8 Gy were 0.4 and 0.2 mL (range, 0–2.1 mL); lumbosacral lesions' mean and median cauda equina doses were both 10 Gy (range 2–14 Gy), and the mean and median cauda equina volumes exceeding 8 Gy were 0.64 and 0.5 mL (range, 0–2.9 mL). These were doses to the spinal cord or cauda equina from the radiosurgical treatment only, not composite doses that included the contribution from prior conventional RT (given to the majority of the lesions) (18). Among 86 patients in the Henry Ford Hospital's experience who survived longer than one year, only one was observed to have myelopathy, which occurred at 13 months following radio-surgery. The average spinal cord volume defined at the treated spinal segment was $5.9 \pm 2.2$ mL. The Henry Ford group had escalated the prescribed dose as their experience evolved; in patients who received 18 Gy as the prescribed dose, the 10 percent of spinal cord volume receiving the highest dose (i.e., the hottest 10 percent of spinal cord volume) had received an average of $9.8 \pm 1.5$ Gy. The spinal cord volume receiving greater than 80 percent of the prescribed dose was $0.07 \pm 0.10$ mL ($1.3 \pm 1.8$ percent of the spinal cord volume defined at the treated spinal segment). Regarding the single patient with myelopathy, she had been prescribed 16 Gy, and her spinal cord dosimetry was modest in comparison to that of other patients (the 10 percent spinal cord volume dose was 7.6 Gy, and the maximum point dose to the spinal cord was 14.6 Gy) (20). No patients in the Memorial Sloan-Kettering experience were observed to have myelopathy (19). Benzil et al. treated 31 patients, with 35 lesions, most with metastatic lesions, but this group also included nine primary tumors (four intradural, five extradural), and dose schedules were variable. Two patients experienced radiculitis, but their symptoms were transient (16). Gibbs et al. treated 102 lesions in 74 patients, with prior conventional RT in two-thirds. The radiosurgical dose schedules were variable (16–25 Gy in 1–5 fractions, with a dose-per-fraction of 7–20 Gy). Neurotoxicity was observed in 3 patients, without significant recovery, and two of them were noted to have had anti-angiogenic or epidermal growth factor receptor inhibitor therapy within two months of developing clinical injury (15).

As most patients who undergo spine radiosurgery are patients with metastatic cancer and short life expectancy, the current state of the art in terms of treatment-associated myelotoxicity is acceptably low. However, it is possible that patients with longer survival potential are at higher risk for myelotoxicity; this patient group includes those with treatment-responsive or indolent metastatic cancers and those with nonmetastatic, primary spinal tumors, which might not limit life expectancy. In this regard, the Stanford experience with radiosurgery for spinal cord arteriovenous malformations is instructive, as the radiosurgical target was the intramedullary spinal cord lesion per se. Fifteen patients were treated to an average dose of 20.5 Gy, given over 2–5 fractions (thirteen patients received 20–21 Gy in 3–4 fractions, and two patients received 20 Gy in 2 fractions). No neurologic toxicity was observed, and the mean follow-up interval was 28 months (21).

## Accuracy in Terms of Patient Immobilization and Treatment Delivery

The target in spine radiosurgery is always in close proximity to the main avoidance structure, the spinal cord. Therefore, radiosurgical treatment plans have steep dose gradients, such that even small errors in patient positioning can inadvertently bring the spinal cord into the high dose region. Guckenberger et al. examined actual spine radiosurgery treatment plans and simulated translational and rotational positioning errors. Translational errors in the transverse plane were found to have the greatest effect on spinal cord dosimetry. To keep the dose to the hottest 5 percent of the spinal cord volume to within $\pm 5$ percent or $\pm 10$ percent of the prescribed dose, errors in the transverse plane would have to be no greater than 1 mm or 2 mm, respectively (for longitudinal positioning errors resulting in the same spinal cord dosimetry variances, maximal translation was found to be 4 mm or 7 mm, respectively) (22).

A number of patient immobilization devices have been described for spine radiosurgery. At Memorial Sloan-Kettering Cancer Center, serial CT scanning was used to demonstrate that positioning accuracy was generally within 2 mm with either one of two systems: a stereotactic body frame (which uses pressure plates applied to the anterior and lateral pelvic bones, lateral ribs under the arms, and sternum) or a body cradle, which uses a vacuum mold (19,23). However, a few patients were found to have transverse translational errors as large as 5 mm (19). Positioning errors of similar magnitudes have been found by other investigators (24,25).

Verification imaging modalities used for positioning verification once a patient has been placed in the immobilization device have commonly included localization X-ray films and infrared optical tracking (12). Recent advances in image-guidance have provided the ability to perform CT scans of the patient once on the treatment machine, either by using the linear accelerator itself to generate the CT image (26) or by using a conventional X-ray tube mounted orthogonally to the linear accelerator gantry (27). These image-guidance methods permit repositioning of the patient on the treatment machine prior to treatment delivery.

# References

1. Patchell RA, Tibbs PA, Regine WF, et al. Direct decompressive surgical resection in the treatment of spinal cord compression caused by metastatic cancer: A randomised trial. *Lancet* 2005;366(9486):643–648.
2. Rades D, Stalpers LJ, Veninga T, et al. Evaluation of five radiation schedules and prognostic factors for metastatic spinal cord compression. *J Clin Oncol* 2005;23(15):3366–3375.
3. 8 Gy single fraction radiotherapy for the treatment of metastatic skeletal pain: Randomised comparison with a multifraction schedule over 12 months of patient follow-up. Bone Pain Trial Working Party. *Radiother Oncol* 1999;52(2):111–121.
4. Hartsell WF, Scott CB, Bruner DW, et al. Randomized trial of short- versus long-course radiotherapy for palliation of painful bone metastases. *J Natl Cancer Inst* 2005;97(11): 798–804.
5. Wu JS, Wong R, Johnston M, Bezjak A, Whelan T. Meta-analysis of dose-fractionation radiotherapy trials for the palliation of painful bone metastases. *Int J Radiat Oncol Biol Phys* 2003;55(3):594–605.
6. Wai MS, Mike S, Ines H, Malcolm M. Palliation of metastatic bone pain: Single fraction versus multifraction radiotherapy: A systematic review of the randomised trials. *Cochrane Database Syst Rev* 2004(2):CD004721.
7. Sze WM, Shelley MD, Held I, Wilt TJ, Mason MD. Palliation of metastatic bone pain: Single fraction versus multifraction radiotherapy: A systematic review of randomised trials. *Clin Oncol (R Coll Radiol)* 2003;15(6):345–352.
8. Schultheiss TE, Stephens LC, Jiang GL, Ang KK, Peters LJ. Radiation myelopathy in primates treated with conventional fractionation. *Int J Radiat Oncol Biol Phys* 1990;19(4): 935–940.
9. Schultheiss TE, Stephens LC, Ang KK, Price RE, Peters LJ. Volume effects in rhesus monkey spinal cord. *Int J Radiat Oncol Biol Phys* 1994;29(1):67–72.
10. Ruifrok AC, Stephens LC, van der Kogel AJ. Radiation response of the rat cervical spinal cord after irradiation at different ages: Tolerance, latency, and pathology. *Int J Radiat Oncol Biol Phys* 1994;29(1):73–79.
11. Philippens ME, Pop LA, Visser AG, Schellekens SA, van der Kogel AJ. Dose-volume effects in rat thoracolumbar spinal cord: An evaluation of NTCP models. *Int J Radiat Oncol Biol Phys* 2004;60(2):578–590.
12. Jin JY, Chen Q, Jin R, et al. Technical and clinical experience with spine radiosurgery: A new technology for management of localized spine metastases. *Technol Cancer Res Treat* 2007;6(2):127–133.
13. Hristov B, Shokek O, Frassica DA. The role of radiation treatment in the contemporary management of bone tumors. *J Natl Compr Canc Netw* 2007;5(4):456–466.
14. DeLaney TF, Park L, Goldberg SI, et al. Radiotherapy for local control of osteosarcoma. *Int J Radiat Oncol Biol Phys* 2005;61(2):492–498.
15. Gibbs IC, Kamnerdsupaphon P, Ryu MR, et al. Image-guided robotic radiosurgery for spinal metastases. *Radiother Oncol* 2007;82(2):185–190. Epub Jan 24, 2007.
16. Benzil DL, Saboori M, Mogilner AY, Rocchio R, Moorthy CR. Safety and efficacy of stereotactic radiosurgery for tumors of the spine. *J Neurosurg* 2004;101 Suppl 3:413–418.
17. Gerszten PC, Burton SA, Ozhasoglu C, Welch WC. Radiosurgery for spinal metastases: Clinical experience in 500 cases from a single institution. *Spine* 2007;32(2):193–199.
18. Gerszten PC, Burton SA, Belani CP, et al. Radiosurgery for the treatment of spinal lung metastases. *Cancer* 2006;107(11):2653–2661.
19. Yamada Y, Lovelock DM, Yenice KM, et al. Multifractionated image-guided and stereotactic intensity-modulated radiotherapy of paraspinal tumors: A preliminary report. *Int J Radiat Oncol Biol Phys* 2005;62(1):53–61.
20. Ryu S, Jin JY, Jin R, et al. Partial volume tolerance of the spinal cord and complications of single-dose radiosurgery. *Cancer* 2007;109(3):628–636.

21. Sinclair J, Chang SD, Gibbs IC, Adler JR, Jr. Multisession CyberKnife radiosurgery for intramedullary spinal cord arteriovenous malformations. *Neurosurgery* 2006;58(6): 1081–1089; discussion 1081–1089.
22. Guckenberger M, Meyer J, Wilbert J, et al. Precision required for dose-escalated treatment of spinal metastases and implications for image-guided radiation therapy (IGRT). *Radiother Oncol* 2007;84(1):56–63.
23. Yenice KM, Lovelock DM, Hunt MA, et al. CT image-guided intensity-modulated therapy for paraspinal tumors using stereotactic immobilization. *Int J Radiat Oncol Biol Phys* 2003;55(3):583–593.
24. Lohr F, Debus J, Frank C, et al. Noninvasive patient fixation for extracranial stereotactic radiotherapy. *Int J Radiat Oncol Biol Phys* 1999;45(2):521–527.
25. Ryu S, Fang Yin F, Rock J, et al. Image-guided and intensity-modulated radiosurgery for patients with spinal metastasis. *Cancer* 2003;97(8):2013–2018.
26. Mahan SL, Ramsey CR, Scaperoth DD, Chase DJ, Byrne TE. Evaluation of image-guided helical tomotherapy for the retreatment of spinal metastasis. *Int J Radiat Oncol Biol Phys* 2005;63(5):1576–1583.
27. Jaffray DA, Siewerdsen JH, Wong JW, Martinez AA. Flat-panel cone-beam computed tomography for image-guided radiation therapy. *Int J Radiat Oncol Biol Phys* 2002;53(5): 1337–1349.

# Index